SKIP THE GUILT TRAP

SIMPLE STEPS TO HELP YOU MOVE ON WITH YOUR LIFE

GAEL LINDENFIELD

To Stuart, my husband, who has been the most wonderfully supportive partner to have beside me when I needed to pull myself out of a guilt trap, or just to have a good laugh with about the fact that I had slipped back in there again!

Thorsons
An imprint of HarperCollins*Publishers*
1 London Bridge Street
London SE1 9GF
www.harpercollins.co.uk

First published by Thorsons 2016

10 9 8 7 6 5 4 3 2 1

A catalogue record of this book is available from the British Library

ISBN 978-0-00-814436-4

Printed and bound in Great Britain by Clays Ltd, St Ives plc

Contents

Introduction

Guilt is not a bad feeling any more than love is a good feeling.

If we do bad things in response to either feeling, we are likely to be in trouble.

If we do good things in response to either feeling, we are likely to be rewarded.

If we do nothing in response to either feeling, we are likely to become trapped by emotion and depowered.

To some people these statements may seem obvious, but it took me many adult years to be able to say them sincerely. From early childhood I was terrified of guilt. It wasn't so much the fear of hell fires that caused my terror; it was the fear that I would never become a saint. That had been my burning ambition from as far back as I could remember.

So as a child I seriously strived to be so pure that I would never feel guilt. But however many good conduct badges I earned, I still did. At that time, I belonged to a religion that required me to confess all my sins before receiving Holy Communion. Not only was it expected of me to receive this sacrament, I wanted to do so. I knew it gave you grace and that was what I needed in abundance to become a saint. When the time for confession approached, I would panic. I felt guilty about not having any guilt to confess! My solution was to invent some sins just so I had something to say to the priest. One of those was, of course, lying. I hoped that God would understand.

When in my late teens I stopped believing in God, my guilt problem didn't disappear. I started to do things that 'should' have made me feel guilty but didn't. So then I was back once again to feeling guilty about not feeling guilty!

Unsurprisingly for a wannabe saint, I drifted into the helping professions. There, I found that I was certainly not alone with my problem. In fact, I was spending a good deal of my working days trying to persuade others not to feel so guilty.

Eventually, I decided that I needed to get a firmer grip on the issue of guilt. I could see that it was causing innumerable kinds of relationship and mental-health problems. I started researching and experimenting with strategies for dealing with this feeling. When I reached a point where I felt confident enough to write a book on the subject, I took the idea to my publisher. A contract for *Triumph Over Guilt* was signed. That book was never written because my younger daughter was killed in a car accident. Guilt once again became a major personal issue for me.

Over twenty years later I have now written this book. I believe it takes a more kindly approach to the subject than my first synopsis did. I now appreciate more fully the positive aspects of guilt. In contrast, over this period guilt has been categorised by psychologists as a negative emotional state.[1] It appears that many other mental-health professionals are also concerned about the increasing negative impact this feeling is having on people's mental health. But my aim in writing this book is still the same as it ever was. Above all, I wanted to write an easy-to-read, USEFUL book that could be used as a self-help programme by someone on their own or with a small group of friends.

Is this a book for me?

- **Yes**, if you are someone struggling with guilt issues in <u>everyday life</u> situations such as:
  – losing your concentration because you still feel guilty about the mistake you made last time you tried that same task;

– when faced with a difficult decision, you think, *Well, I know I'll be damned if I do and damned if I don't;*
– obsessively looking over your shoulder to see what others are doing and wondering if you are doing it right;
– when a relationship ends you can't stop thinking of what you wished you had done that might have made it work;
– when someone has died and you find it hard to move on because you feel guilty about enjoying life when they are not around;
– being a parent who says and does things that you regret and who keeps on thinking that you might have damaged your child or their chances forever;
– feeling so guilty about being happier or richer or more successful than others around that you cannot enjoy what you have;
– feeling constantly bad about not being able to look after someone in the way you think you should;
– dwelling on things you wish you could have done differently in your childhood;
– feeling bad about something you did in the past but have not owned up to;
– feeling partly responsible for something that went wrong when others were accused and punished and you were not;
– having cheated and now regretting your actions;
– being a survivor of a disaster or serious illness when others were not so lucky;
– if you feel guilty about hurting others by your own life choices;
– if you feel guilty about not feeling guilt!

- **Yes**, if you would like to become clearer about when you should feel guilty and when you should not.
- **Yes**, if you would like to just check that you are dealing with guilt in a confident and assertive manner.
- **Yes**, if you want to help anyone else handle their guilt more effectively.

And also,

- **Maybe yes**, if you have been treated for a mental illness in which guilt has played a part and are now on the road to recovery. This book should help to handle any future guilt in a constructive and self-affirming way.
- **Maybe yes**, if you have committed a crime and been punished but still feel guilty. But it would be advisable to work through this book with the support of someone who is a professionally trained psychotherapist or counsellor.

How to use this book

I suggest that you first read this book through quite quickly. You need not bother with the exercises or to practise the strategies now, but do mark up the parts of the book that you think could be useful for you. It would also be good to note down any examples of situations in your life that you have found difficult as they come into your mind when you are reading.

On your second reading, do the exercises and try out the strategies as you go, taking special care with the ones that you have marked. Again, make notes as you go along. After this reading, it could be very helpful to discuss the book with one or more of your friends. This might help to jog your memory and feel less alone with your problem.

Finally, make a prioritised list of issues that you want to resolve or work on. Then return to Chapter 9, Guilt into Goals, and do an action plan. Don't forget to try to find a supportive person to help keep you on track.

Over the next few months, keep the book in a handy place where you can consult it whenever you need to. Having it lying around at home may encourage others to dip in and start wondering if this is something that may help them as well.

I do hope that you will find the book interesting and stimulating to read. I also, of course, hope that it will help you to move on with your life more happily and confidently.

CHAPTER 1

What Exactly Is Guilt, and What Is the Point of It?

Psychologists call guilt a *'self-conscious'* emotion. Other emotions in the same category are pride, embarrassment and shame. All these emotions differ from our basic emotions such as fear, disgust and joy, which are more instinctive and universally felt during the first year of our lives. Self-conscious emotions develop later when we begin to get a sense of ourselves as separate from others. This usually occurs towards the end of the second year and through the third year of our lives.[2]

Before we can feel guilt, we must be able to make judgements. This can't happen until the thinking centre of our brain (the neocortex) is sufficiently developed. This means that babies and very young children *cannot* feel guilt. Their brains are simply not well enough developed to process it. Physiologically, they cannot understand the difference between right and wrong.

At thirteen months, my little granddaughter sometimes appeared to know when she had done something not allowed. She would throw her food on the floor and look at us with a big grin on her face. This was not because she enjoyed being wicked (that will come later!). Her smile had been generated because she was enjoying seeing the reaction of us adults. And perhaps because we were still in the honeymoon phase of grandparenting, we found her behaviour funny and so would laugh along with her. Unsurprisingly, she would then instantly repeat it without the slightest hint of guilt!

However, this guilt-free phase of life is all too short. I was recently taking a walk along a fairly deserted beach when I came across two little naked girls at the edge of the sea. When they spotted me one of them hastily stood up and placed her bikini pants over her private parts. Although they were giggling and smiling, I noticed that their heads were bowed. My guess is that they were around three years old, the age at which guilt starts to creep its way into our psyches. Fortunately for them it had not yet developed well enough to spoil their innocent enjoyment of being 'naughty'.

This pleasurable stage in guilt's development is one that many adults often try to recapture. Here are some examples you might recognise:

- Girls' days out in health spas where groups of gym-toned, professional women get drunk on champagne and greedily devour forbidden desserts.
- Boys on get-fit golf breaks, egging each other on to have yet another drink until dawn appears.
- Carnival participants dressing up in outrageously shocking costumes and singing songs that in everyday life would not be tolerated.
- Office parties where people let their hair down and the next day return to work smiling but with their heads down, just like the little girls on the beach.
- Buying food and drink labelled guilt-free, while being aware that they may still be far from nutritious.

On a more serious note, some people simply cannot feel guilt at all. Early in my career I used to work on the locked wards of a large psychiatric hospital. Many of our adult patients had a reduced capacity to reason. Through disease or arrested development, the centres of their brains that are used to process guilt were not functioning. As a result, much of their behaviour would have appeared to the outside world as selfish, anti-social and excruciatingly embarrassing. Because they were incapable of feeling guilt, I – along with other members of staff – had to learn to accept and tolerate their behaviour. It was a good lesson to learn so young, because since then I have met many adults and young children in the outside world who are also incapacitated in this way.

What's the point of guilt?

Guilt, like other self-conscious emotions, probably emerged in our human evolutionary development at the time when humans started to form groups. They did this in order to work and protect themselves from enemies more efficiently. The function of the self-conscious emotions was probably to make these groups stronger by encouraging loyalty and self-discipline. Anyone who has set up or led a group will know how important these two qualities are. Basic emotions such as fear and anger can be used to encourage or enforce discipline only up to a point. After a while they induce resentment and rebellion. Guilt, on the other hand, encourages self-control. We keep to 'the rules' because we don't want to feel it. The pain induced by guilt is internal and therefore not as disruptive to the rest of the group as, for example, anger might be.

This is how we think nature first intended guilt to work. Note that nature has a back-up plan if Plan A doesn't work (always an excellent idea!).

NATURE'S ORIGINAL PLAN A FOR GUILT

A group member breaks a written or unwritten group rule:

- The thinking centre in their brain assesses that they have done wrong and sends an alert to the emotional centre of their brain.
- They feel guilty.
- They assume responsibility for the wrongdoing.
- They are motivated to either repair any damage their wrongdoing may have caused, or to leave the group.
- The wrongdoer is either integrated back into the group or forgotten, and business carries on as usual.

NATURE'S ORIGINAL PLAN B FOR GUILT

A group member breaks a written or unwritten group rule:

- On feeling guilt, they don't follow through with Plan A. They don't own up, and they don't make things right.
- The other members or the group leader notice the body language of guilt (e.g. perhaps that give-away bowed head).
- The person is accused and either punished or expelled.
- The wrongdoer is either integrated back into the group or replaced, and business carries on as usual.

Of course, we all know that nature's plans (like our own) do not always work. If they did for guilt, I wouldn't feel the need to write this book! But it is important to remember that, in its essence and when well managed, guilt is a good and useful emotion for both the individual and any group to which he or she belongs. It is there to ensure the healthy survival of the group. This is why positive guilt is one of ten categories of guilt that I have chosen for us to discuss and work on in this book (see Chapter 2).

At some later stage in human development individuals began to formulate their own moral codes. At first, their personal rules for living a 'good' life would be shaped to a large degree by their country's culture and laws. But today, in our global world, people are also internalising moral influences through travel, the Internet and the media. The problem is that this ad hoc absorption of so many differing philosophies, religions and laws has sent our moral compasses spinning. We either feel guilty about whatever course of action we take, or we give up on guilt because we think, *I'll be damned if I do and damned if I don't.* The psychological effect of this moral confusion is bad news for the individual's mental health and bad news for any group or society to which they belong.

The good news, though, is that you will find many of the tips and strategies in this book will help with these tricky contemporary moral issues.

The difference between guilt and shame

These two emotional states are often referred to interchangeably in everyday language. It doesn't help the confusion that they are also often experienced together. But there are some important differences between them. The simplest explanation of the difference that I have heard came, surprisingly, from a comedian:

Guilt is feeling bad about what you have done; shame is feeling bad about who you are – all it is, is muddling up things you have done with who you are.

MARCUS BRIGSTOCKE, BRITISH COMEDIAN

But if you wish to have a more academic evaluation, Christian Miller from Wake Forest University, USA, did an interesting summary of the differences that have been found by researchers.[3] Below, I have selected a few of the points she made that are relevant to our work in this book. Remember, these are only some of the differences that have been found through research.

- Guilt is a private emotion, whereas shame usually develops as a result of disapproval – real or imagined – from others.
- Shame can be triggered not just by moral wrongdoing, but by failing to abide by certain laws, rules or usual etiquette that do not have a moral base, e.g. wearing the wrong kind of dress to a wedding, forgetting to brush your hair before going to work or failing an exam.
- Guilt relates to wrongdoing that has been done. Shame concerns how you feel about yourself. You don't like yourself at all, or you don't like an aspect of yourself, rather than you don't like what you have done.
- Shame makes you feel helpless, but guilt doesn't always do so. In fact, guilt often prompts you to try to make amends or makes you wish that you could. Shame makes you want to hide yourself away so you and your failures are not noticed.
- When we are ashamed, we are less likely to feel empathy with anyone else who might have suffered as a result, e.g. people who put a lot of time and money into helping us with a project that we failed to deliver. With shame, we might be feeling so sorry for our failings that we cannot feel sympathy for anyone else who has suffered. With guilt, our focus might be on how we have let people down.
- Guilt is more likely to make us want to get into action to help others in some way. Shame doesn't do this because it makes us feel useless.

As this kind of information always makes more sense when we apply it to our own personal experiences, try this exercise:

EXERCISE: CLARIFYING THE DIFFERENCE BETWEEN GUILT AND SHAME

The purpose of this exercise is to help you judge which aspects of your response to a past wrongdoing indicate whether you were feeling shame and/or guilt. Being aware of roughly to what degree you felt each emotion will help you to decide the kind of action you need to take. As you know, this book is largely about dealing with guilt, but we will also deal with one kind of guilt that has a large element of shame mixed in with it. I call this Shameful Guilt. My two examples here illustrate how a wrongdoing can trigger both emotions.

Think of a time when you felt guilty and/or ashamed and ask yourself these questions:

a) Did I feel that I wanted to hide away or did I want people to know how bad I felt?
b) Did I do something that was morally wrong or not (as opposed to just breaking a rule or law that many people think is daft or out of date)?
c) Was my focus primarily on myself or on others?
d) Did I feel bad because I had done something ethically wrong (e.g. *I wish I hadn't done that*) or did I feel bad that others would judge me as stupid/inept/inadequate/too ugly, etc. (e.g. *I'm such an idiot*).
e) Did I do something to repair my wrongdoing or did I do nothing?

Using a scale of 1–10 (10 being the highest amount for either feeling), score yourself separately on the amount of guilt and/or shame that this aspect of your response indicates you were feeling.

Example 1

Wrongdoing: *I was unnecessarily cruel to say what I said in that meeting – he was only a trainee. I was so shocked by my behaviour that I was speechless.*

a) a) I only wanted to hide away. I didn't consider acknowledging my guilt to others.
Shame 10/10 Guilt 0/10

b) Morally, I was totally in the wrong. The trainee was trying and I was unnecessarily aggressive about his naïve suggestion.
Shame 0/10 Guilt 10/10

c) My focus was largely on myself – I hardly thought of what he must be feeling.
Shame 8 /10 Guilt 2/10

d) I knew what I had done was very wrong, but I was more worried about how others would judge me.
Shame 9/10 Guilt 5/10

e) I didn't even apologise.
Shame 10/10 Guilt 10/10

Example 2

Wrongdoing: *I lied to Mum in my message. I told her I had to work all weekend. I just couldn't face driving all the way there – she's such hard work these days. But I did worry about her and rang her on Sunday for a chat.*

a) a) I told Jim what I had done but wouldn't have told anyone else.
Shame 7/10 Guilt 2/10

b) Jim said stop worrying, it was only a white lie. But I do think lying is wrong and I could have just told her that I was exhausted. Not going to see her every weekend is not that selfish – I do go often.
Shame 5/10 Guilt 3/10

c) My focus was largely on Mum.
Shame 0/10 Guilt 7/10

d) I was largely concerned about whether what I had done was right or wrong in relation to my own values. I was also slightly concerned about what Mum would think of me.
   Shame 1/10 Guilt 9/10
e) I did make good enough amends.
   Shame 0/10 Guilt 9/10

Repeat this exercise two to three times for other occasions when you felt guilty and/or ashamed.

As you continue reading this book, repeat this exercise and think of other occasions when you felt guilty and/or ashamed. It might help to have some photocopies of the exercise ready to fill out. By the time you have finished the book, you should have become an expert on the differences between these two emotional states.

What does guilt feel and look like?

Most of us think we know the answer to this question. We will readily describe what we feel inside our bodies and how it makes us behave. But your personal experience may be different from what others feel. People notice and describe the 'signs' of guilt in different ways. They may also behave differently. To confuse us even more, many of the signs of guilt can be due to other causes. So we may have to rule these out first before we can be confident that they can be attributed to guilt. But the lists that I am going to give you below are a good clue as to whether or not guilt *could* be at the root of a problem.

Here are some of the ways different people have tried to describe their personal experiences of guilt:

How different people experience guilt

IN THE BODY

There's a permanent knot in my stomach.
It's like pain and sorrow mixed with each other.
I feel like I want to cry but can't.
I go quiet – it's as though my throat has tensed up and I can't speak.
It's like a bunch of moths eating at my insides.
I often feel like I am going to be sick.
I want to hit my head … and I often do!
I find myself hitting my leg as soon as I remember it.
I want to curl up in a ball and my body starts to do that.
I feel scared and go all jittery.
I have this tension in my head – and I just can't get my body to relax.
I want to hide – my head bows and my eyes close.
I feel like I am carrying bags of lead weights.
My head feels like it weighs a ton.
There's like a weight on my heart.
It's like I can't stop sighing.
It's weird … sometimes I just feel dirty and that I need to wash and wash … Perhaps I'm going mad, like Lady Macbeth!

IN THE MIND

It makes me think that I should not have done what I did because everyone else thinks it is bad.
I feel like my mind is going to explode.
I go over the situation again and again in my head.
I think people may be talking about me – thinking I am bad or am doing something wrong.
Thinking again and again of what my father would say if he could see me now.
I always think I am making a mistake.
I keep having flashbacks to when it happened.
I am constantly thinking that I should have done it differently, even though others are pleased …
Telling myself if only I had worked just that bit harder I could have …
It's like I keep thinking that I will be 'found out'.

I keep imagining what could have happened if I hadn't been lucky.

Sometimes I feel guilty about being alive ... I just can't get it out of my mind that others died through no fault of their own.

Constantly telling myself I was such an idiot.

I can't get the thought out of my mind that life isn't fair – why have I got everything I have when others can't? Just the luck of the draw.

I just worry all the time that I am getting it wrong and should know better.

It feels as though I am an impostor at work.

I just find myself dwelling on the fact that I could have done more ... even though I really know I did what I could at the time.

Sometimes people are not aware that they are feeling guilt. When they first come to me, many of my clients may experience some of these 'symptoms' and think they are due to ill health or external stresses. If the latter have been ruled out, we will then look together at how they have led and are leading their lives. This is when it is helpful to also know what the common behavioural signs of guilt are, which may be the underlying cause of distress.

In the next chapter we will be examining in some depth the different types of guilt and the behaviours associated with each. But for the moment here are some of the more common general signs of possible guilt that you may recognise:

Behavioural signs of guilt

- Avoiding certain people or all people, or subjects of conversation.
- Playing too safe.
- Overcompensating with extremely 'good' behaviour.
- Overwork.
- Obsessions.
- Depression (without an obvious cause and no bipolar disorder diagnosed).
- Agoraphobia.
- Dependence on alcohol or drugs.
- Rebelliousness.
- 'Bad' behaviour.

EXERCISE: MY PERSONAL SIGNS OF GUILT

- Re-read the lists of physical, mental and behavioural signs that I have given above, and mark the ones that you commonly experience.
- Ask a couple of people you know what they feel and notice in their mind and behaviour when they feel guilty. You could show them the lists above. Note the differences in your experiences of guilt.

Who is more likely to feel an unreasonable amount of guilt?

Although there is no definitive research that can prove the cause of this problem, there are some reasons that are commonly accepted among therapists and counsellors as to why some people feel excessive or unreasonable levels of guilt. Below, I am listing the main ones that I have come across in my own work. Having an idea of how a problem started or was encouraged (and maybe still is) can help us to identify possible ways to deal with it.

We are more likely to get caught in a guilt trap if we:

- are generally known to have an emotionally sensitive temperament;
- are introverted;
- did not have enough love given or shown to us in our childhood;
- were 'outsiders' or considered to be 'different' in our family or childhood institutions and became resigned to being so;
- as children were bullied or have been repeatedly so in adulthood;
- were brought up in an overly disciplined family or institution;
- have spent a long time in a highly disciplined and authoritarian profession;
- have lived a long time in a politically repressive society;
- have been members for a long time of a social group with a very strict ethical framework;
- belong to a group that has strong moral directives;

- belong to a religious group that does not encourage interaction with people of other beliefs or faiths;
- have chronic low self-esteem;
- do not have a secure idea about the kind of person we are or want to be;
- are perfectionists;
- are not good at standing up for our own rights;
- still feel the need for parental approval;
- never like to rock the boat and almost always strive to keep the peace;
- do not currently have a strong supportive network.

On reading this list you may have noticed that I did not include any gender issues. Although I often hear and read the opinion that women feel more guilt than men, to my knowledge there is no research to back up this belief. Women perhaps talk more openly in everyday life about their guilt. Men do not do this so much, but will drink, overwork or bash a boxing bag to reduce the tension, but then suppress it. However, in the confidential confines of therapy, I see little difference between the genders. Certainly the causes appear similar, as does the degree of distress.

EXERCISE: HOW PREDISPOSED AM I TO GETTING CAUGHT IN A GUILT TRAP?

1. Re-read the above list again. This time do so more slowly, giving yourself time to think about each characteristic. Mark the ones that have some significance for you.
2. Discuss with members of your family or a friend.
3. Make some notes.

Summary

- Before we can feel guilt, the neocortex regions of our brain must be fully functioning and we must able to:
  a) understand the difference between the concepts of right and wrong;
  b) learn and remember that there are standards that others may expect us to meet or that we ourselves may want to meet;
  c) be self-aware enough to notice the sensations that we experience when guilt has been triggered.
- Guilt has evolved along with other self-conscious emotions to strengthen groups by encouraging loyalty and self-discipline.
- Guilt and shame are different. Guilt is a feeling we have when we think we have done something wrong. Shame is what we feel when we think we are a bad person because we have done something wrong.
- We may each feel guilt in different ways, even though some of the signs of guilt may be shared.
- Some of us are more predisposed to get caught in a guilt trap than others.

CHAPTER 2

Ten Different Types of Guilt

We often hear guilt described in oppositional terms such as 'healthy'/'unhealthy' or 'rational'/'irrational'. I confess to having talked about it in these terms many times myself, and I still do occasionally. But the reality is that people who have difficulty in managing guilt are usually experiencing a messy muddle of a number of types of guilt, including both oppositional kinds. And to make matters worse, people's inner cauldron of guilt is forever changing.

As we can't see or touch feelings, naming and describing the problem we have with them is very helpful. It makes the issue more real and is an important first step towards dealing with it. Furthermore, if we see it in black and white outside our head, our thinking brain becomes top dog, rather than our emotional brain. We can then often see clues as to what we may need to do to manage the problem better. This is not just true for us as individuals; it also applies to groups, organisations and societies, too.

So I have compiled a list of the ten most common types of guilt that I have encountered. I will describe each kind and give you some examples. This should help you to identify the types of guilt that trouble you, and understand the kinds that other people you know may experience.

Please remember that my ten types do not constitute an exhaustive list. If you don't feel your guilt fits under any of these categories, try creating one or more new labels and write a short description for each. I am confident that you will be able to apply the advice and strategies in this book with minimal adaptation.

Positive guilt

As we noted in the last chapter, guilt evolved in humans as a helping mechanism. For those of us whose experience with guilt has been quite negative, it is important to remember that it can still be very good for us, and also for the world we live in.

When guilt is felt **appropriately**, and the wrongdoer feels the **motivational** urge to make **recompense** and then takes **constructive action**, it has the power to be positive. Let's look at a couple of examples:

1. Ian had a journey from hell coming back from work. When he arrived home, his six-year-old son jumped on him to greet him. Ian irritably brushed him aside. On seeing the tears well up in his son's eyes, he felt a surge of guilt. He immediately took his son in his arms and said he was sorry. He then asked if he could make up for his bad temper by having a kick-around with him with his new football. His son was delighted!
2. Janine was newly appointed as a manager in a store. Her brief was to improve the turnover. This was her first management post and she had been told by her boss that she would now have to 'toughen up' her style of relating to her team, many of whom had become her friends.

   For the first six months she tried and failed. Turnover didn't improve and she became alienated from her colleagues. She knew that she was doing something wrong, but she didn't know what. Her staff were obviously demotivated and Janine felt guilty and concerned. She decided to try a weekend course in interpersonal skills that she had seen advertised in her store's newsletter.

The course was enlightening and helped her to see that her style of management had been aggressive and was having a demotivating effect on her staff. She was recommended an eight-week evening assertiveness training course and decided to do it.

> **Hard though it may be to accept, remember that guilt is sometimes a friendly internal voice reminding you that you're messing up.**
>
> MARGE KENNEDY, NOVELIST AND PLAYWRIGHT

At work the next day, she called a meeting of her staff and told them what she had done and intended to do. She apologised and asked for their help in giving her honest feedback while she was trying out a better style of interacting with them. The end result was that morale improved enormously, and so did the turnover.

Ian and Janine's examples show that positive guilt can be beneficial not just to us, but also to others. It can also be used for the **prevention of wrongdoing**. This is particularly so if it is used in conjunction with empathy. Here's a simple example of good parents using it well:

Twelve-year-old Joe is kicking up a fuss about having to go to his grandmother's birthday tea. Instead, he wants to spend the afternoon with his friend. His mum tells him his gran will feel very hurt and disappointed if he doesn't go. She adds, *'I know how much you love your gran, so wouldn't you feel guilty if you hurt her feelings?'*

Of course, some might argue that Joe's mum may be using guilt in a manipulative, controlling way here. But let's assume that she isn't, and that she is simply using it to help her son become more empathic and kind.

There are many other different examples of anticipated guilt being used positively as a preventative aid. Instilling a sense of loyalty is a powerful way of getting people to conform of their own free will. It motivates people to keep 'in line' and avoid the guilt they would feel if they let the side down. Additionally, it doesn't provoke the resentment that formal authoritarian power can induce.

Leaders of all kinds use the 'threat' of guilt to **build loyalty** within their staff or team members.

- CEOs will create values-based mission statements and urge their employees to live up to them.
- Sports coaches will motivate their teams by reminding them 'not to let the side down'.
- Soldiers are regularly told that being part of a battalion is an honour, and to *'stand by your mates whatever'*.
- Actors are fed the message that for the sake of the audience and the other actors *'the show must go on'*, however tired or hungover an individual may be.
- Card manufacturers and social networks encourage us to keep our personal support systems alive by sending caring messages saying *'Thank you'*, *'Get well'*, *'Good luck'* and *'Congratulations'*.

Anticipated guilt is also used more directly to **encourage helpful behaviour**. For example:

- donor cards sitting by shop tills and medical reception counters;
- the rattling of charitable donation tins in full public view;
- *'Smoking harms others'*, *'Drinking and driving kills'* and Neighbourhood Watch scheme posters.

All these examples give our positive-guilt buttons a gentle push. Sometimes, however, guilt buttons need a stronger push to transform them into a positive force. Interestingly, a series of research studies done by Stanford University in the United States, led by Professor Francis Flynn and Becky Schaumberg, revealed a strong correlation between guilt proneness and leadership. Guilt-prone members of the research group seemed to the rest of the participants to be making more of an effort than the others to ensure everyone's voice was being heard, to lead the discussion and generally to take charge. Even when they did the test in a real-world setting, a strong link emerged between a participant's guilt proneness and the extent to which others saw the person as a leader. Becky Schaumberg reported that these guilt-prone people showed the most responsibility. They were prepared to lay people off in order to keep a company profitable, even though they felt bad about doing so.

> **... the most constructive response [to making mistakes], and the one people seem to recognise as a sign of leadership, is to feel guilty enough to want to fix the problem.**
>
> PROFESSOR BECKY SCHAUMBERG, STANFORD UNIVERSITY[4]

Is it any wonder that leaders tend to use guilt frequently to push or pull the people they lead?

Finally, it is important to remember that for guilt to work positively, there does need to be an element of caring involved. For example:

- **The people involved are part of a group who love or respect each other** such as a family, friendship group or team of close colleagues. Miguel, a star footballer, went out on a drinking binge to celebrate his brother's birthday. It was the night before a big match and the match was lost. The coach had noticed that Miguel had not been performing anywhere near his best. When he confronted him, it was obvious that Miguel felt more than usually gutted and quickly confessed what he had done. He expressed his guilt to his teammates, apologised profusely and asked for their help to stop this happening again.
- **The guilty party has empathy with the victim's suffering** and cares enough about them to want to make amends. Sometimes this empathy may have to be induced

to prompt a caring feeling. For example, a ten-year-old boy had stolen from another child at school. The teachers arranged for him to meet with his victim and hear about how the boy felt and the difficulties that the theft brought him.

- **The guilty party cares about the goal that has been mutually agreed and is still mutually wanted.** When Carole had an affair, she and her husband Bob agreed to stay together and try to make it work for the sake of the children. A year later Bob started an affair himself. Six months later, his fourteen-year-old son uncovered his secret. Bob didn't feel bad for his wife, but he did feel guilty that he had not been careful enough to hide it from the children. He broke off the affair and committed to couple counselling with his wife.

> **Every man is guilty of all the good he did not do.**
>
> VOLTAIRE

Summary: Positive guilt

- If guilt is a justified response to some real wrongdoing and motivates the wrongdoer to take constructive action to repair the wrong, it is positive.
- Anticipated guilt can be used positively to strengthen and motivate individuals and groups of all kinds.
- Pressing our positive-guilt buttons can encourage us to be more empathic and helpful.
- If we are prone to guilt, we could make a good leader.

Suppressed guilt

This is the kind of guilt that occurs when someone is aware of the feeling but consciously keeps it hidden inside, although it does then have a habit of surfacing into the mind from time to time. This can happen without any obvious prompting, but more frequently a reminder will trigger it. The person may well intend to do something about their guilt one day, but as time goes on they find this harder to do. So their guilt grows, and then they beat themselves up for procrastinating. The longer they leave it, the harder it becomes to deal with.

Nothing is more wretched than the mind of a man conscious of guilt.

PLAUTUS, ROMAN PLAYWRIGHT

Over the many years since my daughter Laura's death at age 19 in a car accident, I have had quite a number of emails, cards and letters expressing this kind of guilt. They have come from a range of people, including many of her friends who were her age at the time.

Most have said similar things: they have often thought of Laura and felt bad that they had never expressed to us what she meant to them. They have then told me about the qualities they appreciated in her and how much they missed her. They have apologised for not letting me know this earlier, when others did come to see me and send cards. They say, or imply, that they have felt guilty ever since. What a shame that they were unnecessarily troubled internally for so long with this bad feeling. Their 'wrongdoing' was so understandable and forgivable.

Festering inner guilt does our mental health no favours. It eats away at our self-esteem and makes us more prone to anxiety. It can also cause people to behave in inappropriate ways. For example, a person who is having (or has had) an affair will often take out their tension on the family whom they love and don't want to desert. Or they may do the opposite and overcompensate by spoiling the children and even the spouse they are cheating on.

The longer we leave suppressed guilt locked away, the harder it can be to confess and deal with. Firstly, the wrongdoing can become less forgivable by the victim, even though they may appear to have moved on.

Secondly, by the time the wrongdoer is ready to deal with it, the chance that trust and respect can be established between the parties has probably diminished greatly.

> **I was tormented with guilt for years and years. In fact, it was so bad that if I didn't feel wrong, I didn't feel right!**
>
> JOYCE MEYER, AMERICAN AUTHOR

Thirdly, after a very long period even sensible people can suddenly get a now-or-never urge to confess or apologise. By then, their overwhelming emotional need is so strong that they can make a clumsy or inept attempt to talk to the victim. Here's a sad example:

A well-known and internationally respected person recently confessed on the radio that she felt bad about the way she had run away from home some twenty-five years ago. She hadn't spoken to her parents since. She found out that they were due to travel from a certain airport and decided to go there. She found their check-in queue and went up to them. She wasn't recognised, so she told them who she was. They greeted her politely and then walked on, and she hasn't seen them since. How very, very sad.

Then fourthly, an overdue 'outing' of guilt often causes the victim's and their supporters' thirst for revenge to be intensified. This can lead to inappropriate and sometimes cruel punishment. Recently, for example, a number of court cases have taken place in our country against people who committed seriously dreadful crimes over 40 years ago. Several were given prison sentences, even though they are now in their late eighties and nineties and are seriously ill. Mercy was not considered an option, even when remorse was expressed.

> **There is only one way to achieve happiness on this terrestrial ball, and that is to have either a clear conscience or none at all.**
>
> OGDEN NASH, AMERICAN POET

Finally, the torment of suppressed guilt, especially when the above problems have been witnessed in others, can lead to these attitudes: *I will be damned if I do, so I might as well not try*, or more scarily, *I'll be damned if I do, so I might as well be even more evil or die.*

In Chapter 7 I will be suggesting some more effective ways for dealing with suppressed guilt.

Summary: Suppressed guilt

- Suppressed guilt is the kind that is consciously felt, but is not outwardly expressed.
- It damages the mental health of the guilty person.
- It can have knock-on negative effects on the people with whom they interact.
- The longer the guilt is suppressed the more difficult it is to deal with and there is a risk that the consequences of outing it will be more negative.

Disguised guilt

This is guilt that has been suppressed, but the person feeling it is not currently consciously aware that they feel guilty. It becomes apparent only because of other mental-health symptoms or other problems. The mental-health symptoms can vary enormously from classified illnesses such as depression, OCD (obsessive-compulsive disorders) and addictions. The other problems may be more everyday issues such as persistent relationship difficulties, career issues, low confidence or anger mishandling. It is during the investigation of possible causes of these problems that buried guilt is uncovered as a contributing cause. Traditionally, and probably most commonly, this takes place with a therapeutic professional such as a psychiatrist, psychotherapist or counsellor. At the start of consultations clients often say, *'I have no idea why – everything was fine. I have a good job and a great family. The first panic attack came out of the blue. I didn't know what was going on. That started me off getting anxious. I just worry about what to wear, about getting lost, food contamination – you name it and I worry!'*

Alternatively, they could deny they have a problem or lay the blame on others: *'She thinks I've become anti-social and prefer my tablet to people. Yes, I like games, but I'm not addicted – I'm shattered after work and they relax me.'*

Professional therapists are trained to look for hidden causes of problems, especially where there seems to be no obvious reason for symptoms. They are skilled listeners who will focus as much on body language and what is not being said as on what the person is saying. If the cause isn't evident in their present life, they will also take an interest in the person's past as well. In this way they may uncover guilt about a wrongdoing that the client may have completely forgotten about, or not considered relevant to their current issue. Sometimes this guilt is rational and sometimes it is not. Very often it is a mixture of the two.

In my twenties I was diagnosed with serious depression. Luckily for me I was referred to an excellent (and very patient!) therapist. The main reasons for my mental state were plentiful and complex and I don't need to spell all these out now. But it is relevant to share with you how disguised guilt played a part in stopping me from moving forward once my depression had lifted.

Leading up to my depressive illness, I had made myself jobless. I had failed miserably (in my eyes) at two jobs that I had desperately wanted to succeed at. My first was as a childcare officer. One of my clients had beaten his first child so badly that she was taken into care. When the couple had their second baby he and his wife sincerely wanted to make sure that this couldn't happen again. They both adored their new little girl. I visited them regularly and my colleagues and supervisor agreed that they had made great strides in their parenting and stress management. They didn't think it would be necessary to admit the baby to care while I was on holiday. However, when I returned I was told that the father had lost his temper and killed the baby. No one for a moment thought this tragedy was in any way my fault. And in my rational mind I knew that this was true. But my guilt and despair were too great, and I resigned. I vowed to give up social work forever.

After working for some months quite happily as a shop assistant, a friend of a friend told me that a housemother of a children's home was urgently needed. He thought I would be ideal and should apply. As I had spent the majority of my own childhood in children's homes, I was keen to try. And try and try I did. But ultimately I failed. As staff our days were spent stopping the children from beating each other up. The quality care I had wanted to give them, and my staff, was an impossible dream. This time I blamed the system and underfunding and resigned. I felt angry and hopeless and eventually got so seriously depressed that I ended up in hospital.

My psychotherapist cleverly sniffed out guilt as a persistent issue in my troubled history. She unearthed a mountain of forgotten remorse and self-blame dating back to my early childhood. My habitual way of disguising my guilt was to become a rescuer of others. As a child it had started with my kid brother and sister and children weaker than me. By the time I reached adulthood my cause had become global.

As you have probably guessed, this habit is still with me. It is, however, no longer disguised. This means that I can control it and use it in a more focused and constructive way. An added bonus is that this personal experience has left me with a nose for sniffing out buried guilt! Here's an example:

Jeff came to see me because his marriage was falling apart. It emerged that one of the main causes was that his wife thought he had a drinking problem. He didn't accept that his drinking was an issue. He spoke defensively about it and said it was just part of his job. He had to drink sometimes, as that was the way you met and started relationships with new customers.

I encouraged Jeff to tell me a little more about his job. It was one that involved quite a bit of travel. We talked about some of the places he had been to. It emerged that one of them was Budapest. In sharing our impressions of this city he recalled having a one-night stand with a Hungarian colleague. He had virtually forgotten the incident. He laughed it off, saying he was young then and they had both been drinking a little too much that evening. At first he couldn't even remember her name or the year it had taken place, but when we explored it a little more his memory became clearer. As it did, he started to fidget and his hand started covering his mouth. He then recalled that, at the time, his wife had been pregnant with their first child. I noticed that his eyes were looking watery and I quietly asked him how he was feeling. He said, *'Guilty, I suppose, and a bit fearful.'* The fear that he felt was that he would end up like his dad, who was *'a true alcoholic and womaniser'*, and that he, too, might lose his family. He felt immense guilt about not having been able to help his mother more. She remained depressed and bitter until the present day. Jeff was feeling less and less inclined to spend time with her and so feeling even guiltier.

The good news at the end of this story is that Jeff and his wife did repair their marriage. Jeff found new ways to network for new customers and gained a clearer and more rational perspective on his responsibilities towards his mother.

As we know, many people are unwilling to go to a therapist, especially if their problem doesn't feel like a big issue to them. Jeff did, but I don't believe most people need to do so. If the disguised guilt is caught early enough, a partner or close friend who knows the person well may spot it. In Chapter 8 I will outline some guidelines and give some tips on listening in a way that helps people to open up.

Summary: Disguised guilt

- This is guilt that the person is not aware they are currently feeling.
- It can produce emotional and behavioural symptoms that are attributed to other causes.
- The habit of disguising guilt (real or imagined) can often be traced back to childhood.
- The process of outing this kind of guilt needs to be done skilfully and sensitively. A therapeutic professional often does this. Others who know and care for the person can also achieve it.

Childhood guilt

This is a subject that I could easily write a whole book about, and so could most psychotherapists. Childhood guilt is one type that surfaces so frequently. It is one of the main contributing causes of chronic low self-esteem and a host of other common mental-health problems.

As is now common knowledge, our default emotional auto-responses are largely 'wired in' during our childhood years. This makes them much more difficult to control. This is especially so if we experienced guilt repeatedly or it arose as a result of a traumatic experience. Even when, as adults, we can see that many of these responses are not rational and are indeed harmful to us, they still have stubborn sticking power.

Additionally, parents, or other significant adults who had power and influence over us when we were children, induce much of this guilt. Here are a few brief examples of these kinds of 'messages' that I have come across through words, attitudes or consequences:

- You're supposed to be a bright boy; the trouble is that you're just lazy. That's why you failed ... I feel so ashamed of you when I hear this from teachers.
- You'll drive me to an early grave with all that noise. I'm shattered. [From a mother who died of breast cancer in her thirties.]
- Now look what you've made me do. [From a father who had just turned over a table in anger and cut his hand picking up a broken glass.]
- Having to do this hurts me more than it hurts you, but you deserve it. [When being given an overly severe punishment.]
- She's a bully and a liar ... I suppose every family has a black sheep. She's my cross. [Overheard telephone conversation.]
- I told you to watch them ... now look at what has happened. Your brother is in A&E. [Told to an eldest child when she was nine years old.]
- You're going to end up just like your father – you just can't be bothered and think only of yourself. [Father abandoned the family and has been on benefits most of his life.]
- I told you that you looked like a slut in that dress ...What do you expect when you dress like that? [After a 14-year-old had been through an upsetting sexual advance.]

And, of course, damage can also be done indirectly through nobody's fault. I met someone in her eighties recently who, when she found out what I was writing about, said she still feels guilty about her own birth. She was premature and her mother was unable to have any more children afterwards.

Here are some other examples I have known where people feel guilty about being who they were born to be:

- Being born blind, and knowing that his disability has restricted his parents' and siblings' lives.
- Being less intelligent than average and needing private tutoring before all her exams.
- Being more intelligent than her brothers and sisters and getting a scholarship, which enabled her to go to university and have a good career.
- Being a promising sports person whose training and matches have required sacrifices from all his family.
- Being born illegitimate and '... *bringing shame on the family and ruining my mother's life*' (shared by a very elderly man).

And then, of course, there are the guilty secrets that some children felt they had to keep (rightly or wrongly), such as:

- stealing from Mum's purse and Dad's wallet;
- hating a brother the parents favoured and praying he would die;
- lying repeatedly to cover up hurting a younger sister;
- blaming a school friend for doing something you know he didn't do;
- masturbation and other sexual explorations;
- feeling attracted to the same sex;
- missing Dad and secretly meeting him after the divorce;
- going to the synagogue even though they no longer believed;
- lying repeatedly about where they had spent the night;
- being sexually abused by an uncle.

Of course, many people have these experiences and grow up to be able to talk about them or laugh them off. Others unfortunately cannot do this. When they are 'confessed' or discussed, the emotion of guilt visibly floods back into their system. They typically bow their heads or cover their faces with their hands. Unsurprisingly, they commonly feel shameful guilt, which we will be looking at later.

Having guilt from childhood still live within us in adulthood renders us more vulnerable to feeling guilt in the present day. We shall look at ways of dealing with childhood guilt in Chapter 7.

Summary: Childhood guilt

- Many of the behavioural responses that we used to deal with this guilt in childhood become hard-wired into our brains and become our default emotional responses. This makes them hard, though not impossible, to change.
- Parents and other significant adults in our childhood usually induce this guilt, and our relationship with them would have coloured our responses.
- Some of this guilt is no longer relevant to us as adults. It relates to the value systems of other people and not to our own current values. It can, however, still trigger inappropriate responses, which need to be kept under our control.
- Some childhood guilt relates to secret wrongdoing from childhood, which may need our attention because it is affecting our life, relationships or peace of mind today.
- Childhood guilt is often mixed with shame and therefore diminishes our self-esteem.

Parental guilt

Now to the other side of the coin! There cannot be a parent who hasn't been besieged by guilt at some time during their lives. It is a role that the vast majority of us desperately want to do more perfectly than any other we may take on. But, of course, we don't and we can't.

> **I'm trying to avoid, you know, guilt, even though before the child is born you're already thinking you're doing things wrong ... Why do I think that will probably carry over until the day you die?**
>
> EMILY MORTIMER, BRITISH ACTRESS

Once you become a parent, guilt is guaranteed. Nowadays, it even starts nudging us before the baby is born. Recently, I was scrolling through a pregnant mums' internet forum and here are just a few of the 'sins' they were confessing:

- sleeping in the 'wrong position';
- drinking a coffee;
- eating chocolate, Brie and goat's cheese, a fried runny egg and a biscuit that had fallen on the floor;
- drinking one glass of wine in a week;
- moving furniture without asking for help;
- getting stressed at work;
- not doing my yoga breathing;
- not playing classical music for 'the bump'.

After more years than I care to mention, just writing this list managed to trigger guilt in me, too. And that happened, even though in my time we didn't know such 'sins' might harm our unborn babies.

Health professionals with positive intentions induced this guilt. Through leaflets, adverts and face-to-face advice, they pass on the wisdom that has been accumulated from research into pre-natal care. They want mothers to feel guilty if they don't take this new knowledge seriously. When the guilt starts to feel too weighty, most will joke it off in the way they are doing in the kind of forum I mentioned. However, many parents can't do this. This kind of guilt-inducing information stresses them out and frightens them. They can't change the habits of a lifetime overnight.

When the baby is born, that guilt burden will undoubtedly grow. Their pre-natal guilt will leave them predisposed to absorbing more and more. Parental guilt is now a common subject of casual conversation and is regularly addressed in parenting manuals, magazines and websites. But to my knowledge there hasn't been any serious academic research that has proved this rise or pointed conclusively to the reasons for it. From my own practice of working with parents, I have noticed a number of issues that in recent years have kept reoccurring and can cause this accumulation of guilt:

- **Dual careers**. A recent survey by the website Mumsnet.com claims that fewer working mothers are feeling guilty, but now I find that working fathers are adding to the numbers.
- **Financial restraints**. Perhaps some of these are due to lifestyle choices, but many are not. Many people cannot afford to meet their own and their children's needs and expectations. The latter are soaring as globalisation increases and advertising has become so sophisticated. Not so long ago smartphones and individual computers for children were a luxury, but now, when your child's best friend is moving to the other side of the world and they want to keep in touch, and 50 per cent of their class have this year's model, it becomes difficult to say no.
- **Longer working hours**. This may be a problem particularly in the UK where our working hours are extra-long, and it is hard and expensive for families to find quality childcare. Because families are increasingly geographically distant, traditional support is becoming less available.
- **The strains of marital break-up and blended families**. Although these problems are now commonplace, the parental guilt that they trigger seems as high as ever.
- **Rapid rise of mixed-culture families**. This is an exciting development, but it is also challenging for parents. It appears to demand extra commitment, time and negotiation skills. The clash of parenting values and expectations often leaves at least one party feeling guilty about not giving their children the upbringing they believe to be right.
- **The increasing volume of information about childcare available through the internet.** Much of this is good and supportive. However, to unconfident parents encountering difficulties, it can be overwhelming and confusing.
- **The trend that appears to equate a parent's worth with the success and behaviour of their children**. This has become increasingly internalised and parents' self-esteem

and confidence are being affected by this trend, too. This has become an increasing problem as the media constantly confronts us with the images of perfect parents with perfect children. These beautiful images stick and make us wish, '*If only ...*' When parents do seek help, guilt is always the first issue that therapists and counsellors have to deal with before they can move on to their main issues. This is happening in spite of our increasing knowledge of the role that genetic, physiological and cultural issues play in shaping our children.

> **Fatherhood is great because you can ruin someone from scratch.**
>
> JOHN STEWART, AMERICAN SATIRIST

So if it is true that parental guilt is on the increase, it is imperative that we learn how to manage it well. Laughing at it or 'giving up' by slipping defensively into *laissez-faire* parenting brings only very short-term relief and does our children no favours. Almost all the advice and strategies in this book will help. In Chapter 8 there are some tips on how to help children with their guilt, too.

Summary: Parental guilt

- Parental guilt is virtually inevitable for everyone who has a child.
- It arises because parents are naturally programmed to want to do this role as perfectly as possible, and perfection is unachievable for humans.
- It has increased because the contemporary world floods parents with an overwhelming amount of information, which is often contradictory, and due to the stresses of everyday life parental aspirations are often unachievable.
- Parents associate their self-worth today with their children's successes, and this often causes additional guilt. When their children fail or commit a wrongdoing parents are commonly blamed or blame themselves.

Survivor guilt

This kind of guilt was first identified as a special type in the 1960s. It was first applied to survivors of the Vietnam War. But, of course, it did exist before that time, and is now applied to numerous kinds of survival issues. Sometimes it has a rational element and sometimes it does not. Whatever kind it is, it needs to be managed well because it can block sufferers from being able to move on from their traumatic experiences. These are the kinds of thoughts that continually chain survivors to their past:

- I had no right to survive.
- I don't deserve to be here still when they are not.
- If only I had been able to do something differently.
- I should have helped.
- I should have been there.
- It is disrespectful to be happy when they cannot be.
- I shouldn't be successful on the back of their misfortune.

Let's look at some examples of people who have experienced this kind of guilt. These brief quotes illustrate how it can occur in a wide range of life situations and at any stage of life.

I felt guilty for years that maybe I should have run back and tried to get her to stay with me. Maybe I didn't do enough to stay together. Maybe I was too selfish about saving myself.

JOSEPH, HOLOCAUST SURVIVOR

I have started to experience what I can only describe as survivor guilt. Some of my classmates were also good candidates and had similar grades, but they didn't get a place. I have also heard about people who have applied loads of times and they didn't get in either.

FERN, AN 18-YEAR-OLD GIRL IN HER FIRST YEAR OF A POPULAR UNIVERSITY COURSE

I felt so bad about being among the few that didn't get made redundant. I still haven't made contact with anyone to see how

they are getting on, so the guilt is getting worse. No one expected this crash, but perhaps we should have done.

ALAN, AN INVESTMENT BANKER

He may have walked away with his life, but he has been haunted by survivor's guilt ever since.

RELATIVE OF PETER, WHO WAS ON A PLANE THAT CRASHED, KILLING HIS FATHER AND 69 OTHERS

Mum, it should have been me. At least I have had more life.

MY 21-YEAR-OLD DAUGHTER AFTER HER 19-YEAR-OLD SISTER DIED IN A CAR CRASH

He couldn't get past it, he felt really guilty and he kept saying it should have been him that died.

SISTER OF A SOLDIER WHO WAS FOUND HANGED AFTER RETURNING FROM THE AFGHAN WAR AFTER HIS TWO BEST FRIENDS DIED

I did not feel survivor's guilt until two years or so after my bone-marrow transplant. It took me another six months to finally pick up the phone and call my doctor to ask if other bone-marrow transplant survivors ever had these dark feelings of depression and guilt (although I would not have recognised it as guilt).

A 47-YEAR-OLD MAN WHO SUFFERED FROM LEUKAEMIA AND HAD A TRANSPLANT

The soldiers I've talked to involved in friendly-fire accidents that took their comrades' lives didn't feel regret for what happened, but raw, deep, unabashed guilt. And the guilt persisted long after they were formally investigated and ultimately exonerated.

NEW YORK TIMES WAR REPORTER

A dozen decisions that I made over the course of a two-month period could have been wrong but that didn't occur to me at the time. Any one of those made differently may have saved his life. I am still dealing with the guilt of having cost him his life.

A RETIRED ARMY OFFICER TALKING ABOUT THE ACCIDENTAL DEATH OF ONE OF HIS SOLDIERS

All this recent unveiling of sex abuse in the past has made me think back to my own schooldays. There was a history teacher who I am sure was dodgy. He invited me a couple of times to his flat for some extra tuition. He started being different with me – friendlier, putting his arm round me. I didn't go back. Now I am haunted by the faces of the boys who did – they were quite shy. I should have said something.

MAN IN HIS SIXTIES WHO HAS STARTED TO FEEL GUILTY ABOUT NOT RAISING THE ALERT ABOUT A TEACHER AT HIS SCHOOL

Would you believe that I still get pangs of guilt about my twin Peter. I wonder if he would have made a better job out of his life than I did. My parents so much wanted a son and she couldn't have any more after our births.

A 77-YEAR-OLD FRIEND OF MINE WHOSE TWIN DIED SOON AFTER SHE WAS BORN

Most of these people did, of course, move on with their life after their trauma. But many will have suffered with their survivor guilt for longer than they needed to. There are some tips on how to help anyone with similar issues in Chapter 8.

Summary: Survivor guilt

- Survivor guilt was first identified as a condition in the 1960s and for a long time was just applied to people who survived war traumas and felt guilty about living when others died.
- Nowadays it is increasingly accepted that anyone can feel this guilt if they have survived a major trauma of any kind while others were less fortunate.
- This guilt can seriously block sufferers from moving on with their lives.

Affluence guilt

This kind of guilt is about feeling uneasy with having a comfortable lifestyle while others do not share that privilege. It has become an increasing challenge for people in developed parts of the world. The media constantly broadcasts images of those in pain and poverty. Financially strapped charities are now quite understandably using powerful advertising techniques to turn the knife into the consciences of those who are better off.

I know that a man who shows me his wealth is like the beggar who shows me his poverty; they are both looking for alms from me – the rich man for the alms of my envy, the poor man for the alms of my guilt.

BEN HECHT, AMERICAN AUTHOR

Cheap travel has also let many more people see for themselves the contrast between their lives and those of people in less-developed countries. The latest global financial crisis has also brought many face to face with the hardship of others. We don't need statistics to tell us that, in spite of all the aid programmes, the gap between the poor and the rich has widened.

Of course we need to face these uncomfortable facts, but we also need to remember that affluence guilt can become a burden to bear. When this happens we can lose the will to aid those whom we wanted to help. When people become depressed by their guilt they can sink into cynicism or powerlessness.

This tragically ironic quote from John Lennon says it all.

Guilt for being rich, and guilt thinking that perhaps love and peace isn't enough and you have to go and get shot or something.

JOHN LENNON, WHO WAS SHOT AND KILLED IN HIS FORTIETH YEAR

There are many people who would argue with me that the very opposite of affluence guilt is starting up. They might point to the incredible queues that I, too, have seen outside designer shops in some of the poorest countries. They might also draw my attention to the 'canonisation' of celebrities and the way they are worshipped. They would say that their expensive clothes and wealthy lifestyles are emulated rather than criticised.

> **I feel bad sometimes that I ever did it.**
>
> JOHN SYLVAN, A MULTIBILLIONAIRE, ON THE GROUND COFFEE CAPSULE HE INVENTED

Ultimately, everyone has to choose which of these positions to take. The choice will affect the amount of guilt they carry themselves and notice in others. I know it is a subject that troubles many of the people I meet and encounter via the media.

But you don't need to have billions before you feel this guilt. It has been a lifelong issue for me. My childhood experiences undoubtedly were a major influence.

As I have mentioned before, for much of my childhood I was brought up in poorly funded children's homes. From an early age I was aware that I was more deprived than the children around me at school. However, the nuns who schooled me kept me aware of others who were worse off than myself. When I had to choose a saint's name for my first communion, I chose Elizabeth. This saint was a noble lady who was beatified because, in spite of her mean and aggressive husband, she found 'miraculous' ways to help the poor. Throughout my childhood I prayed to this saint to help me become like her. Although during my life I have worked for and given to charities, I have never been able to match her and I never will. No wonder I continually battle with affluence guilt!

> **At this time my only guilt comes from having to charge for the work I do, otherwise I can't put a roof over my head!**
>
> FRANCESCA, A TRAINER AND DEDICATED VOLUNTEER

The tips in Chapter 7 are based on those that have helped me and many of my clients to manage this guilt, which I hope I will never be without.

Summary: Affluence guilt

- Contemporary life presents a constant and often overwhelming stream of information and images of people who are less fortunate than those in affluent, developed countries.
- Charities are using increasingly sophisticated means to nudge the public's conscience, but most people have only limited amounts of money and time to donate.
- Some people are programmed by childhood influences to be more vulnerable to this kind of guilt.

Carer's guilt

This is the guilt we feel when we know we should be caring more effectively for members of our family or others who feel like part of our wider family. The latter could be a friend or neighbour, or a colleague with whom we have a special emotional connection. It is a condition that is now widely acknowledged in most developed countries. Generally, it is applied to people who have members of their family in need of extra-special nurturing and attention because they are unable to manage well on their own, usually because they are elderly or sick or have a disability. There are others – some pregnant mothers, for instance – who may have a temporary need for extra help.

Like most of the guilt types we have discussed, carer's guilt does appear to be on the increase. For centuries, women have traditionally taken on the role of carer within families and communities, but in contemporary society this is no longer necessarily the case – most women have careers as well as families that make heavy demands on their time. In addition, we are living longer and needing more care in our old age. Improvements in medicine have also meant that sick younger people are being kept alive when only a few years ago they would have died.

The most recent change in society that has affected this issue and is a constant feature of media attention is that the quality of care given by the state and private institutions seems to have deteriorated. Regardless of whether or not the scare stories we hear are misleading or unrepresentative, our overall impression is that institutional care is best avoided. This has triggered even more guilt in those who have no alternative other than to put their loved ones in a home.

> **Carers will always feel guilty – it's part of being a good carer and feeling that there is always more that we can do.**
>
> ALZHEIMER'S SOCIETY

Everything I have learned from working with carers myself and from the organisations who currently support carers has convinced me that guilt feelings are inevitable. This is because, as a carer of someone in need, we will always feel guilty when we:

- leave them;
- say no to them;
- begin to feel resentful;
- snap at them because we are so tired and stressed;
- have to leave them with someone they don't know;
- see them look sad or hear them beg us to stay;
- forget to ring them or check up on them;
- learn that they are ill and think we should have noticed;
- see other carers who appear to be doing so much better than us;
- know we are neglecting our family and friends;
- are less effective at work and take time off in crises;
- don't have enough money to give them a better life;
- recall something we did or didn't do that hurt them in the past;
- start to feel sorry for ourselves;
- take time to give ourselves some nurturing or treats.

Our aim must not therefore be to eradicate carer's guilt completely. We need to rid ourselves of the irrational stuff and learn helpful strategies and techniques to manage the inevitable rest. You will find some tips in Chapter 7.

Summary: Carer's guilt

- This is guilt we feel when we think we should be caring more effectively for people in our lives who have a reduced capacity to look after themselves.
- Women have traditionally taken on the role of carer, but as most now work they cannot necessarily do this any longer.
- Through the media we are being made increasingly aware of the inadequacies of institutional care and the rising tide of people who are dependent.
- A certain amount of guilt is inevitable for every carer.

Shameful guilt

I've got the Jewish guilt and the Irish shame, and it's a hell of a job distinguishing which is which.

KEVIN KLINE, AMERICAN ACTOR

We have already looked at the difference between guilt and shame in Chapter 1. Shameful guilt is simply a combination of two kinds of guilt. We feel it when we have done, or think we've done, something wrong and also have a sense that this proves that we are intrinsically bad or not as good as other people. It therefore attacks our inner confidence, which is the bedrock of our mental health. The consequences of feeling shameful guilt are bad for us, and often bad for others as well, because we may:

- not own up to what we have done, or think we have done, because we don't want even more people to think we are bad;
- feel less inclined to apologise, because we believe that they won't want to listen to us;
- not believe someone who says they have forgiven us and wants to wipe the slate clean;
- not make amends for what we have done because being bad means we will probably do it again;
- go on to do even more and possibly worse deeds because that's what people as bad as us do;

- consciously or unconsciously seek out the company of people who are as bad as us;
- become cynical and very negative in our thinking;
- isolate ourselves or not allow people to get too close for fear that they will discover who we really are and the bad things that we are capable of doing;
- start to 'worship' people whom we believe are better than us, and allow that to blind us to their failings;
- become a 'rescuer' of others to the extent that we neglect ourselves in order to be regarded as 'good';
- become very religious, because only a higher power can forgive us;
- become overly self-obsessed and introspective, and so have less empathy with others;
- become depressed and suicidal;
- not seek help because we are worthless and/or others are more deserving.

You may have noticed that some of the possible consequences above are contradictory to each other. This is because shame and guilt are essentially different emotions and have different effects. They can therefore pull you in different directions. So, unsurprisingly, shameful guilt is the most difficult kind to both feel and overcome.

This may also be why it is used to exert power and influence over people. Throughout history, dictators and politicians have used shameful guilt as both a threat and a punishment.

Lead the people with administrative injunctions and put them in their place with penal law, and they will avoid punishments, but will be without a sense of shame. Lead them with excellence and put them in their place through roles and ritual practices, and in addition to developing a sense of shame they will order themselves harmoniously.

CONFUCIUS, CHINESE PHILOSOPHER

Teachers were also using it in the days when they put the dunce cap on children, and still do when they make children answer questions in class they know they will get wrong. Even parents use it; for example, when they tell their seven-year-old child in public that they're behaving like a three-year-old.

Inducing shameful guilt is also one of the techniques that advertisers use to sell products. Sometimes they will use it in a direct way by showing, for example, pictures of people with zits on their face or without deodorant looking isolated within a crowd, or indirectly by showing people using their products being super happy and successful. Political parties will also employ advertisers who use shameful guilt to win elections or get people to change their views or behaviour.

But not all of those people using this kind guilt for influence have bad intentions. Many are trying to help people or make the world a greener or safer place. They use this method because it works. But, of course, there are mental-health consequences of doing so for many people. The shame will stick, for example:

- if they can't buy what is suggested as being good for their children, the environment or public health;
- if they cannot conform because the message conflicts with their religious or other deeply held beliefs;
- if they are already too depressed or overwhelmed by another psychological issue to be capable of change.

When shame sticks it can cause all the problems we have already looked at. When it is mixed with guilt it is even more difficult to shift, as Paul Ekman explains.

The distinction between shame and guilt is very important, since these two emotions may tear a person in opposite directions. The wish to relieve guilt may motivate a confession, but the wish to avoid the humiliation of shame may prevent it.

PAUL EKMAN, PROFESSOR OF PSYCHOLOGY, UNIVERSITY OF CALIFORNIA

Many of the techniques and tips in this book will help with this type of guilt, but if you suffer greatly from it you may need extra help as well. It is notoriously difficult to shift when it is well set in. This is especially true if it was first absorbed during childhood and has been reinforced continually throughout many adult years. People feeling a mass of shameful guilt put up invisible barriers around themselves, saying, *'Don't get too close.'* If you try to praise, love or care for them, they will feel worse because they 'know' that they are undeserving. In some cultures shame is believed to be so bad that it is better to be dead than to feel it.

> **Shame is worse than death.**
>
> **RUSSIAN PROVERB**

You could use scripting to ask confidently for help (pages 90–94), and in my Further Help section on page 213 there are some agencies and websites that you can contact. Shameful guilt is one that should be given high priority, because it has the power to undermine us at any time.

Once shame touches your being at any point, even the most distant nerve is implicated, whether you know it or not; any fleeting encounter or random thought will rake up the anguish and add to it.

STEFAN ZWEIG, AUSTRIAN AUTHOR

Religious guilt

This particular form of guilt is the last in my list of ten. It has been placed in this position because, although I am not a professional expert on the subject, this kind of guilt has had a major impact on me as a person and on the lives of many of my clients.

I'm an Irish Catholic and I have a long iceberg of guilt.

EDNA O'BRIEN, IRISH NOVELIST

For most of my childhood I was schooled, like the writer Edna O'Brien, by Irish Roman Catholic nuns. Anyone who knows anything about Catholicism will understand why religious guilt was a central force in my childhood. To be fair, it was a force that by and large kept me on the straight and narrow. And I am truly grateful for that. In particular, I thank the people who insisted on weekly trips to the confessional. These made me stand back from my life and regularly reflect on the morality of my behaviour. It's a habit that has stuck, even though I am no longer a believer and don't use a religious confessional. As an adult, however, I do habitually choose to read novels, see plays and listen to radio debates that centre on moral dilemmas. Like my trips to the confessional, this habit serves to challenge my own moral integrity. It has also influenced the way I work as a psychotherapist and without a doubt it has fed my motivation to write this book.

Religious guilt has, however, also brought me and many of my clients and friends a great deal of unnecessary pain. For example, it gave us the burden of guilt inherited from distant ancestors. The Catholic concept of original sin gives all its adherents a heavy dose of guilt with which to start their lives. But they are not alone. Other religions do the same. There are those who are told that their reason for being in the world is that they did something so wrong in a past life that they had to spend this one atoning for it. And nowadays, as religious fanatics exert violence on our contemporary world, we are being reminded of how our ancestors behaved similarly in the name of religion.

Religious tenets and practices learned during childhood become so ingrained that, even when they are rejected in adulthood, lingering ghosts remain.

SUSAN CARRELL, AUTHOR OF *TOXIC GUILT*

These kinds of 'messages' feed a foundation of ready-made religious guilt into our collective psyches. This renders us more generally attuned to guilt. So when something bad does happen, the default response in many of us is to feel guilty and try to think of what it is that we have done wrong.

Occasionally something good, such as useful understanding, will emerge from this introspection. More often than not, though, it just causes stress. In emotionally vulnerable people this can tip them into mental ill health. They will often begin to ruminate repetitively on their guilt, whether it is rational or irrational. At best, this worry will make them tense and anxious, but at worst it can lead to clinical depression or an OCD disorder.

Because I now work in London, which is an international city, I frequently see people who are in mixed-religion partnerships. They may have chosen to consult me with regard to their low confidence, but religious guilt often emerges as one of the causative factors. They have rarely felt able to discuss the matter with members of their family. Joseph, a young doctor, was an example. He was referred to me for help with his lack of confidence. It had been said that it would affect his chances of obtaining a promotion. It emerged during our talks that he was deeply in love with a Christian English girl. He was hiding this relationship from his parents.

There is no way that I could bring it up. I have to marry into the faith. My mother would be devastated and my father would probably kick me out of the house. I don't want that, and anyway I can't afford it yet. [He gave a 'naughty child' smile as he said the last sentence.]

JOSEPH, A 24-YEAR-OLD JEWISH JUNIOR DOCTOR FROM IRAQ

Fortunately I was able to help Joseph in the first stage of tackling his problem. We looked at ways to rebuild his inner confidence. He was good on the outer skills, but was quaking inside. We rebooted his self-esteem and he learned some strategies to help him think more positively. We then worked on how best to communicate his situation and fears to his parents. (You will learn how to do this yourself in forthcoming chapters.)

The religious guilt issues that have been most frequently shared with me have been between parents and teenagers. Usually it is the parents who are religious and the teenager who is questioning or rebelling. This is an age-old generational problem, but since the rapid growth in fundamentalism I think it is eliciting more fear, particularly in parents.

Recently I bumped into an ex-client at an airport and we had a coffee together. I talked about my project – this book – and she said:

My parents were very religious. They were such GOOD people and did so much charitable work. As a child I was also very

religious and loved going to church. When I left home I stopped. I didn't stop believing in God, but religion just wasn't that important. A book I read recently started me thinking and pricking my conscience. I have been a couple of times to one church since, but I didn't feel it was for me. I think I should be part of the church, but I'm so knackered after work. I have started to feel very guilty about letting my parents down as well as God.

ADEL, A 47-YEAR-OLD WEST INDIAN TEACHER FROM BIRMINGHAM

Knowing Adel, I am guessing this prick to her conscience will lead to a positive outcome. Her self-esteem is in good shape and she is already doing valuable work at her school and in her family life. I don't think it will be long before she finds a church community that does suit her, and her guilt will quickly diminish.

Like me, others may choose to look for more secular solutions when their religious consciences are feeling unsettled. I am hoping this book may help some of them. I have tips to try in Chapter 7.

If only I wasn't an atheist I could get away with anything. You'd just ask for forgiveness and then you'd be forgiven. It sounds much better than having to live with guilt.

KEIRA KNIGHTLY, BRITISH ACTRESS

Summary: Religious guilt

- Even people who have given up their religion can suffer with this guilt, especially if religious influences were strong in their childhood years.
- Religions use guilt as a motivator for good behaviour and also to keep people under their influence.
- Today's multiculturalism has helped to increase this guilt, because it forces many people to make decisions about the way they live which are not in harmony with their religious beliefs.

CHAPTER 3

The Four Key Personal Qualities That Will Help You

1. Self-esteem

Here are two facts that it is crucial to get stuck fast in your mind now, and forever!

1. If you are prone to feeling guilty, you will also be prone to low self-esteem.
2. If you are prone to low self-esteem, you will also be prone to feeling guilty.

Maybe these facts make instant sense to you already. But if they don't, I hope they will by the end of this section. We have already examined guilt in some depth, so let's now take a brief look at self-esteem. Then we can begin to look at the relationship between the two in some real-life situations.

Self-esteem is at the heart of mental health and self-confidence. It is what gives us the belief that we can be liked, loved and appreciated for who we are, faults and all. It is also the key inner quality that fires us up to make the kind of success out of our lives that **we ourselves** will take real pride in.

Another plus for high self-esteem is that it is also the bedrock of resilience. Resilience is the ability to pick yourself up and carry on positively after a mistake or setback. It is, therefore, a must for those of us who become trapped by guilt.

When we are stuck in a guilt trap, the best way to start climbing out of it is to give your self-esteem a boost. One of the quickest ways to do this is to focus on changing the language that we use, because much of it will almost certainly be counterproductive. Let's look at how this works with four different people in various real-life situations that have produced guilt.

Firstly, let's look inwards. Even if you haven't been in any of the following situations, I am guessing you will recognise the style of the inner self-talk.

Examples of self-esteem-bashing self-talk

Done it again! How insensitive you can be, you idiot? You've blown it this time. He'll forgive you, but she won't – you don't deserve it.

PAUL – WHO FORGOT IT WAS HIS SON'S BIRTHDAY,
AND BOOKED AN IMPORTANT WORK CONFERENCE AWAY

Why did I shout at her? She's only five years old! She looked terrified. Perhaps she thought I was going to hit her. Of course I wouldn't ... but then maybe I could. I don't know any more. I shouldn't have let her go to school without a hug. She is going to feel really bad all day. What kind of mother am I ...?

FRANCESCA – A MOTHER WHO WAS STRESSED ABOUT GETTING
TO THE SCHOOL AND TO HER WORK ON TIME

I don't even remember turning the alarm off. How could I have gone back to sleep, today of all days? Oh no, I'm going to be over an hour late. He's going to go ballistic at me ... I've screwed it up well and truly this time ... Getting wasted last night was crazy.

ADAM – WHO OVERSLEPT BECAUSE OF A HANGOVER

You should have gone back in ... others did, and firemen do it all the time. And what have you done with your life since? You're

still a gibbering wreck. And you're in big danger of becoming a tranquilliser junkie. Those people in there were doctors and nurses. You're still just a clerk.

GILL – A HOSPITAL CLERK AND A SURVIVOR OF A HOSPITAL FIRE FIVE YEARS AGO

Then, later, if or when guilt is confessed to someone else, their self-esteem will receive a further bashing. This could prove to be even more hurtful and also trigger more guilt:

Examples of self-esteem-bashing responses from others

You didn't forget, did you? ... I can't believe it. What kind of father are you, son? No wonder she's angry – and she's the best thing that ever happened to you. What's up with you? ... You destroy every chance you ever get.

PAUL'S FATHER

You really must get a grip of that temper of yours. Of course you frightened her ... you frighten me. I knew something was up with her as soon as I saw her – she clung to me ... that's why I sat down with her. She said, 'Mummy doesn't like me any more.' That's terrible. No wonder she didn't want a hug from you at lunchtime.

FRANCESCA'S HUSBAND

How could you let me down? ... I gave you a second chance and this is what you do with it ... You're your own worst enemy ... No excuses – I can recognise a hangover when I see one. You look a mess. You're fired!

ADAM'S BOSS

Don't tell me you're thinking about that fire again! I don't want to hear about it. I've heard enough. You have to snap out of it – others have. Look at Sally – she's even got a promotion since. Stop feeling sorry for yourself. I have to get up in three hours for work. Take another tablet.

GILL'S HUSBAND

In the first three examples the guilt was rational and some would argue that the responses from the people in their lives are justly deserved. That may be so, but if these people are ever going to be able to recover from their mistakes and make effective amends they will need to repair their self-esteem.

In our fourth example, Gill's guilt might not have been rational, but it was causing her major problems. Her self-esteem was also undoubtedly damaged and will also have been in need of repair.

Before we move on to how we can repair such damage, let's look at how it could have been prevented. There are better ways of responding to guilt situations that can actually protect and strengthen our self-esteem. The language we use is key.

Firstly, as most people know nowadays, how we talk to ourselves is important. Our self-talk directly affects our mood and shapes the way we think and present ourselves to the world. If it is negative, it will diminish our ability to deal constructively with our guilt.

Secondly, the responses we give to people who, when our guilt is exposed, react negatively is also key. If these are also negative the very relationships that are crucial to supporting us could be seriously damaged.

So, let's look at the kind of language that will be most helpful to your self-esteem in such situations.

Language that will protect your self-esteem when you are feeling guilty

How best to talk to yourself and respond to others' negative responses to your feelings of guilt:

Verbal:

- Make simple, short statements clearly accepting responsibility for what you have, or think you have, done wrong.
- Tell yourself of the positive aspects that are relevant to the situation – especially if these have been ignored or you have been incorrectly accused.

- Apologise if you can, but only once (you can repeat it later, if that apology appears to have been genuinely unheard).
- Share any learning you have gained from the experience.
- State briefly what you intend to do to make amends.

Non-verbal:

- Use a calm, brisk pace.
- Emphasise key words and phrases by slightly pausing before saying them with a firm voice.
- Stand tall while pulling your shoulders back slightly.
- Use direct eye contact to start with and for as much time as you can.

Keeping to these guidelines may seem like a tall order. That's because it is! It is much harder to do than it looks. Even the most confident people find it hard, because guilt is so powerful at pulling us downwards. If you are someone who has been prone to guilt and low self-esteem for a long time, it may take a few months of *repeated practice* to get the hang of using this different kind of approach.

This exercise will give you a chance to apply this theory to one of your own guilt situations. Although it may look long, it should only take you ten minutes at the most to do.

EXERCISE: USING PROTECTIVE LANGUAGE FOR YOUR SELF-ESTEEM WHEN YOU FEEL GUILTY

1. Re-read the examples that I gave earlier in this chapter of Paul, Francesca, Adam and Gill's self-talk, and other people's responses to their guilt.
2. Read the alternative self-esteem-strengthening versions, which I have given below. You will, of course, have to use your imagination to 'hear' and 'see' their body language.
3. Re-read them, but this time notice their key messages and how their revised words and phrases match up with the verbal language guidelines I gave you earlier.
4. Now read these new versions out loud. While doing so, be sure to use the non-verbal language that I suggested above.

5. Note how you feel as you read. Ask yourself what you found okay to say and what was perhaps more difficult. This will indicate where you may need extra practice.
6. Think of something you still feel guilty about. If possible, choose an example that you haven't shared with anyone for fear of how they may react.
7. Imagine that you are going to now confess to that person. (You don't have to do it in real life!) Write down some self-talk to use that will ensure your self-esteem stays intact.
8. Imagine and write down what you fear the other person could say or think in response to hearing of your guilt.
9. Compose a reply using the guidelines that would protect and strengthen your self-esteem.
10. Give yourself a treat!

EXAMPLES OF THE ALTERNATIVE LANGUAGE THAT PAUL, FRANCESCA, ADAM AND GILL COULD HAVE USED TO PROTECT THEIR SELF-ESTEEM (NOTE: I HAVE HIGHLIGHTED PHRASES WHERE THE KEY POINTS ARE BEING MADE):

Paul

To himself:

I forgot his birthday but that doesn't mean I don't love my son. **I do love him** and I will arrange an extra-special birthday treat for him to show him that I am sorry. I will put a permanent reminder in my diary a month before his birthday so that this doesn't happen again. I will explain this.

To his dad:

Dad, I did forget and I am taking steps to ensure that I don't forget **ever again. I *am* a good father**, albeit not a perfect one. I will be making it up to him. Also I love and appreciate my wife and I've apologised and told her what I am doing.

Francesca

To herself:

I shouted at her because I am stressed. I will take some time out to restart yoga. I will buy a book on anger management. I love my daughter deeply and can become **an even better mother**. I will get up 15 minutes earlier so we are less rushed.

To her husband:
I understand you being angry. What I did **was wrong.** I will do everything in my power to deal with my stress and learn to manage my temper better. I am **committed to being a good mother**, as I love my daughter with all my heart. I am so sorry to have upset you as well as her.

Adam
To himself:
I have made a **big mistake**. It has been a major wake-up call. From now on one drink after work is the most I will ever have from Monday to Friday. I now have a **chance of a fresh start** and will make the very best of this.

To his boss:
I fully appreciate why you are firing me. I do deserve it. Thank you for giving me that second chance. This has been a wake-up call for me and I intend to give myself a fresh start. I am **absolutely committed to my career**. There will be **no more** getting wasted during the week for me.

Gill
To herself:
The fire was five years ago and I am still suffering with guilt. It is time now for me to get some help. I will do the exercises in the book. I will also look for a PTSD self-help group or a counsellor if I need extra help. **I am not going to let this guilt destroy my marriage.**

To her husband:
I am so sorry for disturbing you again. It's true that I'm still stuck with this survivor guilt. I've already bought a self-help book, which is helping me. I may also look for a support group and/or a counsellor. **Our marriage is so important** to me that

I would be happy to sleep elsewhere until I feel confident that I have this guilt under better *control.*

> **The saints are the sinners who keep on going.**
>
> ROBERT LOUIS STEVENSON

Now, here are some easier ways to continue strengthening your self-esteem. You could focus on one of them every week for the next couple of months. Some are quick and can be done instantly, others will take a little more time. If you try them all out, you will soon find the kind that works best for you.

Tips for rebooting your self-esteem when you feel guilty

1. **Increase your physical self-nurturing.** This is such a basic way of showing yourself love. Watch caring parents cuddle a child who has done something naughty and is genuinely sorry. Note down seven adult equivalents of giving yourself a 'cheer-up cuddle'. Assign one for each day of the week and test them out, such as a 15-minute break with your favourite drink/listening to your favourite music/soaking in an aromatic bath.
2. **Treat yourself to frequent laughs.** This will help you to keep your guilt in perspective and give you an instant lift. For example, watch short YouTube clips of your favourite comedians in your coffee breaks, or keep regular contact with witty friends with whom you can have some banter.
3. **Give up a bad habit** – for at least one week. (Yes, you may have spotted the ex-Catholic in me! It is like a penance. It does work and you do feel renewed.)
4. **Do something you are good at.** This can be a simple short task. For example, if you are a good listener, phone a friend whom you know could use ten minutes of your time to 'dump' their worries or play a game at which you are both expert.
5. **Reward yourself for something you think you have recently done well or well enough** – and fight against any

sabotaging messages that your guilt might fire into your mind, such as, *You don't deserve it; others did better.*

6. **Write a glowing testimonial for yourself.** You don't have to show it to anyone. Keep it real or it won't work.
7. **Bring an image of a reformed 'sinner' to mind.** This could be someone famous or someone you know: Nelson Mandela, the 'terrorist' who became an icon of political goodness; a rock star who kicked a drug habit; your delinquent brother who became a loving father. The media is full of examples – so no excuses!
8. **Visualise a past moment of pride.** Choose a quiet spot to relax in, close your eyes and recall in vivid detail an occasion when you achieved a goal you are proud of. Feel the pride that you had then and enjoy it now.
9. **Set an inspirational goal for yourself.** Think small, otherwise in the guilty mode that you are in you may set yourself up for failure.
10. **Deepen a special relationship.** This should be someone who loves or likes you and knows you are not perfect. Send them a card, buy them some flowers or just give them a ring to say you miss them.

Finally, you can always give your self-esteem a thorough makeover when you have a little more time to spare. My book *Self-Esteem* is a complete self-help programme for doing just this. I would also recommend two of my other books for many more quick and easy ways to give you a boost: *Self-Esteem Bible* and *101 Morale Boosters.* In this section I have only been able to scratch the surface of self-esteem building. I cannot emphasise enough how crucial it is for you to have truly good self-esteem. It will give you a resistance to absorbing unnecessary guilt. It will also make you less dependent on others' approval and forgiveness so you can stay in charge of your own conscience.

> **Self-esteem and self-contempt have specific odours; they can be smelled.**
>
> ERIC HOFFER, AMERICAN WRITER

2. Humility

> **All streams flow into the ocean because it is lower than they are. Humility gives the ocean its power.**
>
> LAO TZU

At first glance this quality may seem to be contrary to the last one we looked at. I don't believe it is. If we have good self-esteem, we have the confidence to be humble, and this is so necessary if we are to deal well with our guilt and help others deal with theirs. Many successful people have this quality. I have included quotes from some famous people to act as reminders.

I watch *Batman & Robin* from time to time. It's the worst movie I ever made, so it's a good lesson in humility.

GEORGE CLOONEY, AMERICAN ACTOR

What can humility do for us?

It helps us to:

- **accept that we are not perfect** and that neither is any human being. This also makes it easier for us to connect with people from all backgrounds and cultures, which is so important in our contemporary world.

All careers go up and down like friendships, like marriages, like anything else, and you can't bat a thousand all the time.

JULIE ANDREWS, BRITISH ACTRESS

- **confess our mistakes** or express our fear of making them. This is what others want and need us to do, and it will help them to trust us in future.

Humility leads to strength, not weakness. It is the highest form of self-respect to admit mistakes and make amends for them.

JOHN J. MCCLOY, AMERICAN LAWYER AND BANKER

- **ask for help.** You can then make the amends people truly want or need. We can also ask for help with our persistent irrational guilt, which can be very difficult to deal with on our own.

Many receive advice, only the wise profit from it.

HARPER LEE, AMERICAN AUTHOR

- **be genuinely self-forgiving** instead of pleading for forgiveness from others, which they may not want to give. This will help us to stop self-punitive habits. One of mine, like James Baldwin's, was hiding away.

The young think that failure is the Siberian end of the line, banishment from all living, and tend to do what I then did – which was to hide.

JAMES BALDWIN, AMERICAN AUTHOR

- **turn the focus of our thinking more towards others**, especially those we have hurt.

Humility is not thinking less of yourself, it is thinking of yourself less.

C. S. LEWIS, BRITISH AUTHOR AND ACADEMIC

- **ask for critical feedback.** This will help us to avoid mistakes and failures and so prevent unnecessary guilt or worry that we are not good enough.

Take criticism seriously, but not personally. If there is truth or merit in the criticism, try to learn from it. Otherwise, let it roll right off you.

HILLARY CLINTON, AMERICAN POLITICIAN

- **learn from our mistakes.** This is crucial, as this is perhaps the most important step we can take that enables us to let go of both rational and irrational guilt.

If I had to lead my life again, I'd make the same mistakes, only I would make them sooner.

TALLULAH BANKHEAD, AMERICAN ACTRESS

I hope you are now firmly convinced about the virtues of this quality and its relevance to our work. So how do we develop it? As far as I know, no one has yet found a gene for humility. Even if they do one day, I will remain certain that it can be developed from our life experience. This is good news because it means we can take action to strengthen it. Here are some tips to help you do this.

Tips to help you strengthen your humility

Remind yourself of people who have achieved goals that are beyond your capabilities. Read biographies and watch films of extraordinary feats. Listening to interviews with highly successful scientists works for me. (Interestingly for us, you often hear them talking about their mistakes and failures en route to their breakthroughs.)

Keep on studying. Sign up for a class in a skill that you have no real talent for. I did painting and my humility soared!

Share your past mistakes appropriately. Adopt a confident tone and include what you learned from them. *'I once broke a vase of Nana's and I blamed my brother. She shouted at him. I felt so guilty. He was horrible to me for ages and then blamed me for something bigger that I didn't do. I got punished. I learned that it is best to own up.'*

Become an ace questioner. Encourage others to tell you more about what you need to know. Ask people who have moved on open questions that begin with 'what' and 'how', such as: *'I know you said in your talk that you just put it behind you and moved on, but what exactly did you do that helped you to move on? How did you stop the "what if" worries revolving in your head?'*

Invite useful criticism; ask for clarification: *'I know you said I needed to improve, but can you give me some examples of how I could do things differently? I am keen not to make that mistake again'; 'Yes, I accept that I do tend to clam up instead of telling you straight what I am feeling. Can you please tell me at the time when I do this, because it's a habit I don't notice?'*

Let go of your perfectionism in many areas of your life. In fact, in most areas of our lives I believe we only need to do a good-enough job. I can say this confidently as I am a perfectionist, and so are most of my clients. Just keep on regularly asking yourself the question: *'Do I NEED to do this perfectly or would good enough do?'* Ask people close to you to challenge you, too.

> **Humility is a strange thing. The minute you think you have got it, you've lost it.**
>
> E. D. HULSE, BRITISH BARONET AND POLITICIAN

You can, for example, aim for good enough in gardening, home decorating, recycling, home cooking, fitness routines and even parenting. Many of us do, and stay alive to tell the tale!

Don't get complacent about your humility – remember these wise words!

3. Trust

People with a tendency to feel guilt are usually very responsible people. They are driven to do the 'right thing', because they fear getting it wrong so much. That is one of the reasons why they make good leaders. We believe that we can trust them. We are happy to let them look after our interests. We feel safe with them and trust that they won't let us down. They will wade meticulously through information and advice before they make the safest, most effective and most ethical decision. They will also take great care to select exactly the right people to execute the plan. Once they are chosen, they trust that they will succeed and not let the project down. In short, they are inspirational examples of positive guilt.

There are those, however, who have the same good personality drivers, but for some reason their fear of getting it wrong or of others getting it wrong is excessive. Here are a few ways you might recognise them.

THE CONTROL FREAKS

Who:

- become obsessed with planning and organising. Every minute of their 'relaxing' holiday may be scheduled.
- always have to be mega-early for appointments and journeys.
- cannot relax if someone else is doing the driving, even if he or she is a highly trained pilot.
- micromanage anyone who may work for them – breathing constantly down their necks to check every detail.
- are overprotective. 'Be careful' are their favourite words.
- are very nervous of spontaneity.
- find thrill rides their idea of hell.
- know the right way to kick a ball, the best political party to govern, the quickest way to iron a shirt, and even the most efficient way to arrange the contents of the fridge!

How do so-called 'control freaks' become like this? Quite often they have been very hurt by a past mistake and they still feel guilty. They have lost trust in themselves. Sometimes, someone else might have made the mistake or caused the failure, but they may still feel (perhaps wrongly) partly responsible. Commonly, they have some residual rational or irrational childhood guilt, too. The result is that they become overly cautious. Being in control is their way of stopping themselves or others from getting things wrong. They, too, can excel in the right job, but they can become hell to work for and challenging to live with.

In addition, there are those people whose inability to trust others (for similar fear-of-guilt reasons) takes them in a different direction. They become 'rescuers'. Here are some of their traits, which you may recognise.

RESCUERS:

Who:

- appear to be compelled to help others in trouble – even when they may need help themselves!
- feel that they are the best person to help.
- are always chasing their tail. Their diary is full and their phone rings constantly.
- are often on local committees, associations or community groups.
- give to charity even if they are quite poor themselves.
- support causes and often campaign for them.
- never have time for massages or trips to a spa, even though they look very stressed.
- people always seem to turn to for help with their troubles.
- people at work find indispensable, but they don't get promoted.
- get upset when watching disasters on the news, and cry in films that are sad.

They are, of course, good people who are striving to do good things. But again, they can also be pains in many people's necks! This is because they are always stressed, don't ask for help and find it hard to trust anyone but themselves. As they are always noticing the people and situations left in the world that they cannot rescue, their guilt piles up.

In the Western world today, and in many other places, collaborative teamwork and egalitarian relationships are what most people aspire to have. This means that control freaks and rescuers find themselves out of step in their relationships, both at work and at home. They are not in line with either their own or other people's expectations.

I have first-hand knowledge of all these difficulties. I am both a control freak and (as no doubt you've guessed) a rescuer! To compound my problem, I married a man with the same traits! We both had childhoods in which we were let down by people we should have been able to trust. And we were both overloaded with caring responsibilities, which we were too young to take on.

As young adults, both of our first career steps were into social work. Predictably we chose to work in extremely deprived areas, so we felt perpetually guilty for not being able to help enough. In our personal lives, our first marriage choices were bad. We were both deceived over long periods of time – and, of course, we felt guilty about letting that happen!

'*A great match!*' some might say sarcastically. But it was and is! Of course, our guilt and trust issues did need serious attention. Initially, there were many lively battles for top-dog position, and lots of very annoying overprotective habits. These were eventually mellowed by compromise, leaving only minor bickering and a good deal of teasing. And, after 33 years, we still plan to live happily ever after.

In my professional life I have also had many clients with similar guilt and trust issues. So I have learned a good deal about the different ways to handle these. Perhaps the most important knowledge I have gained is that the emotion behind all these trust issues is fear. This is an emotion that you <u>can</u> definitely learn to control (see page 102). For any of you who have similar issues to the control freaks and rescuers, I hope some of these tips will help.

Tips to help you build trust

- Diagnose where your problem originally started. Talk it through with a good friend.
- Ask for 'supervision' from people who could tell you when you are getting into either a controlling or rescuing mode, or appear to be lacking trust.

- When a problem with trust reappears, give yourself some sharp self-talk. Say something like, *I know you are frightened, but you're no longer a neglected kid/living in a war zone/ married to a deceiver/impoverished, etc. You can now control the fear and regain trust.*
- Buy or borrow a book on fear management. Susan Jeffers's *Feel the Fear and Do It Anyway* (Vermilion, 2007) is a classic and would be a good place to start, or you could try my own book, *Emotional Confidence: Simple Steps to Managing Your Feelings.*
- Become a contingency planner. Face your worst-case scenario head on. Always have a plan B and C in case things go wrong. (This is my favourite fear strategy.)
- Join a relaxation or yoga class; do a sport or activity that releases tension.
- Recall a time when you were bossed around too much. Remember how it made you feel. Write it down to commit it to the forefront of your memory.
- Meet and make friends with people who are different from you.
- Play a team sport.
- Join a dance class that involves dependency. (Learning the Argentine tango was testing for both me and my husband, but we did get there eventually!)
- Set off on a holiday without booked accommodation. Too risky? You can take the longest list you want of hotels and guesthouses, but you mustn't book ANY. If you must, make the first trip only 30 miles from your home.
- Count to five before you rush to the rescue.
- Count to ten before you criticise.

4. Empathy

Recently I heard of a newly named psychological condition called 'empathic over-arousal'. I immediately thought, *That's me – that's what I have been suffering with all my life!*

My second, more serious thought, however, was: ... *but I don't suffer*. Yes, my friends, clients and colleagues are right; I do have an unusually high sensitivity to others' emotions, and I do feel their feelings, often very deeply. But I will tell them that they are not right when they assume this must be difficult for me. I have never seen my empathy as a problem. On the contrary, it has always been a bonus. I am glad that my brain's wiring may have given me a head start with this quality. Of course it has proved a big advantage in the job I happen to do, but that is not the whole story. Empathy has immeasurably enriched my personal life as well. More specifically in relation to this book, I know that it has also helped me to deal more effectively with my guilt.

> **You can only understand people if you feel them in yourself.**
>
> JOHN STEINBECK, AMERICAN AUTHOR

The difference between empathy and sympathy

Let's look first at what empathy is. It is the ability to **feel along** with the emotions of other people. When we are with someone who is sharing a problem, we vicariously feel his or her emotion. We may do this consciously or unconsciously. We are **reminded of a time when we experienced a feeling that is the same or similar**. For example:

- I understand. That's just how I felt after my divorce. I was so scared of getting close to anyone again.
- I know you must be so disappointed. It's really hard. I remember feeling just like that when I didn't get the grades for university.

Alternatively, if we are imaginative and very empathic, we can feel along with the other person, even if we have never had that feeling.

- Being mugged like that must be terrible, especially in broad daylight. I've never been mugged, but I have had my car window smashed and been robbed in a crowded street. That felt awful and I was so angry that nobody did anything. But to have been mugged and threatened with a knife in front of everyone must have been so much scarier ... And knowing he still got away ... No wonder you feel angry as well.

- Obviously, I have never lost a child because I haven't yet had any, but I was devastated when I lost my parents within three months of each other. So I have some understanding of what you are going through – you must be so sad.

You can also experience empathy through the **creative arts**. For example, when something bad happens to a character we like in a book or a film, we can react empathetically. A similar experience also takes place when we use creative therapies such as psychodrama. This is a therapy that I commonly use when working with groups. The techniques enable the therapist and participants to stand so well in other people's shoes that they begin to feel like another person and act like them.

People often don't understand the difference between empathy and sympathy, so let me briefly explain what I understand the latter to be. **Sympathy is the reaction we have when we feel sorry for someone in trouble.** Commonly we then offer comfort, reassurance or help:

- It must be very hard to lose a job that you have loved. Do please let me know if there is anything I can do to help. Maybe I can look after the children for you sometimes.

We can also have sympathy for large groups of people suffering from hardship, such as a disaster or poverty.

- Did you see those poor orphans on the news last night? I think I will choose Save the Children as my charity for the marathon.

Empathy's relationship with guilt

Feeling empathy and sympathy is, of course, a good reaction to seeing or hearing of people in trouble. With empathy, however, the quality of our understanding is generally deeper. As such, it makes it more useful in guilt situations.

Firstly, it gives us a better understanding of what the other person may need. This helps us make the kind of apologies they will accept and therefore enables us to make amends more effectively.

Secondly, empathy fuels the 'offender' with more motivation to help. If you are feeling your victim's pain, you want to shed that load as quickly and effectively as you can.

Thirdly, people prefer to take help from those who can empathise rather than just sympathise. The more motivated both parties are in the helping process, the quicker the wounds between them are healed.

Fourthly, empathy also helps us to avoid guilt. It should make us think twice before we do something that might hurt others, or indeed ourselves. This means that when we are drawn towards that delicious chocolate cake in the patisserie window, we will restrain ourselves. We become mindful of how bad all that extra sugar and fat will be for our, our family's and our country's health. A further wag of our finger warns us that if we give in to temptation, we will end up feeling triply guilty!

If you remember, in Chapter 1 we looked at why guilt evolved. It was at a time when nature 'sensed' that we needed some 'social glue' to bond us more firmly into groups. Both empathy and guilt are important ingredients in that bonding mixture. From recent findings in animal biology and neuroscience, we now know that many animals have this 'mixture', too. If you have ever had a dog you will have seen both these ingredients in action. I have had many dogs that felt along with my sadness. They would curl up around my legs or lick my face to show me that they were doing so. Others I remember more for their guilt reactions than their empathy. They would curl into a ball to make themselves look small or slink silently out of the room.

I've learned that some of my dogs, like us humans, were more naturally empathic than others. I wasn't very good at teaching the dogs how to increase their empathy, but I have had better luck with humans! So if your halo has been slipping, here are some tips that could help.

Tips for strengthening your empathy

- **Become more actively curious about people**, especially those whom you may not naturally gravitate towards. Talk to strangers on buses and trains. Relieve queue boredom at airports by finding out where people are going, and perhaps where they wish they were going instead. Sit silently observing people in restaurants and imagining their life. (A bit of discreet eavesdropping is allowed!)
- **Improve your listening skills.** Learn how to encourage the interesting quiet ones to talk, and how to end the conversation if they open up too much (see Chapter 8).
- **Challenge your prejudices.** Try to find commonalities with people you think you dislike – make a beeline for the water cooler when they are there; read revealing interviews and biographies of people who don't share your values.
- **Read more novels and autobiographies** – these are a quick and pleasant way to get to know and understand people of all ages and cultures.
- **Join an arts discussion group.** I belong to four book groups. In spite of the time pressures this gives me, I don't want to give up any. The people, their interests, values and preferred lifestyles are all so different. I confess that also I now like people who, at first, I considered unlikeable. Friends say the same about their film, music, theatre and arts discussion groups.
- **Open up about your vulnerabilities:** share some of your guilty habits and thoughts. Others will then do the same.
- **Use the two-chairs technique** – this is a technique used by psychodramatists and also by actors to help them get into the mind and feelings of a character they have to play. It is not a rehearsal for a real-life conversation.

> **One should examine oneself for a very long time before thinking of condemning others.**
>
> MOLIÈRE, FRENCH PLAYWRIGHT

i. Place two chairs opposite one another. Imagine that you are going to have a conversation with someone you don't understand very well. First, sit in his or her chair. Then, speaking as though you are that person, describe yourself and your life.
ii. Return to your chair and, as yourself, ask the 'other person' a question.
iii. Move to the other chair and answer as them.
iv. Continue having a conversation, moving from chair to chair, until you exhaust the subject – or yourself!

Doing this exercise may feel a little weird at first, but you will soon get into it. I assure you, it is a very powerful technique. (As children, we were once all natural actors. We used play-acting to understand how adults tick – even the wicked ones!)

Read blogs and discussion forums on subjects you know little about. This is free and easy material to look at in spare moments on your phone or tablet.

Study body language. There's lots of free information on the Internet, but also some very good books. Explore these in a bookshop, as the illustrations are important. But don't forget that non-verbal language varies from individual to individual. Experiment with sharing your impressions and asking if you sensed correctly what the other person was feeling – carry on until you get it right most times. Don't worry about getting it wrong – we often learn more when we do! For example:

A) I hope you don't mind me asking. I noticed you frowning and moving your fingers a lot. Are you okay?

B) Yes, I'm fine. I was just trying to remember if we have any fish in the fridge for supper! I often exercise my fingers on journeys. I have early arthritis and want to keep them supple. But thanks for asking. Where are you off to?

Learning to stand in somebody else's shoes, to see through their eyes, that's how peace begins. And it's up to you to make that happen. Empathy is a quality of character that can change the world.

BARACK OBAMA, THE 44TH US PRESIDENT

CHAPTER 4

The Five Key Life Skills

Skill 1: Moral intelligence

No guilt is forgotten so long as the conscience still knows of it.

STEFAN ZWEIG, AUSTRIAN AUTHOR

What is moral intelligence?

The term moral intelligence (MI) has only recently started to be used, so you need not feel guilty if you have never heard of it before! The interest shown in the identification of Emotional Intelligence (EI) towards the end of the 20th century prompted psychologists, academic researchers and educationalists to look at other kinds of 'intelligences'. By the beginning of the 21st century Spiritual Intelligence was also defined and much discussed. The next intelligence to come along was MI. There has been a surge of interest in this in recent years as more and more corrupt practices in the business and political worlds have been uncovered. The repercussions for the organisations have been devastating to their image and finances. So there is now a big interest in how you can identify people with integrity who act in line with moral principles and beliefs without needing to be constantly monitored.

The ideas behind this 'new' intelligence are in fact centuries old. My own interest in this subject dates back to the 1970s when I started training and working in the field of mental health. It soon became obvious to me that this subject was very relevant to the maintenance of good mental health, and in particular to self-esteem and confidence. I hope you will quickly see how applicable it also is to our work on guilt.

The five ingredients of moral intelligence:

Definitions for MI vary considerably, but after reading around the subject and listening to debates for a number of years I have come up with a summary of what I understand it to be.

MI is a collection of the five personal qualities which, when seen in action, indicate that the person has a high level of integrity:

i. Having the mental ability to be able to distinguish between what is right and wrong.
ii. Having a knowledge and acceptance of universal principles that are commonly shared across cultures, such as:
   Integrity
   Responsibility
   Compassion
   Tolerance
   Respect
   Justice
iii. Having the ability to apply these universal principles to **personal values and goals.**
iv. Being able to make decisions in the face of **moral dilemmas and competing desires.**
v. Having the **motivation and will power to behave in line** with universal principles and personal values.

Of course, this outline of MI's ingredients is an ideal. Being imperfect humans, our goal should be, as ever, to reach a good-enough standard. What percentage of the ideal is good enough will vary from individual to individual. As you are reading this book, I am assuming that you are someone who cares very much about values. And that you are concerned about guilt because you want to be a good person and you would like others around you to be good as well.

But I am also guessing that, if guilt is an issue for you, you may not always be reaching what you consider to be a good-enough standard of integrity. There could be all sorts of reasons why this is so. It could be that an overload of stress tempts you to take short-cuts, such as shouting at people instead of encouraging them assertively to get them to do what you want. Or it could be that you have some contradictory values in your head, which means you will never feel you have done the right thing.

People who have high and steady MI rarely get stuck in a guilt trap. This is because their value system is clear to them and it is prioritised. They become aware quickly that they have done wrong. Then they do feel guilt but only briefly. It is a feeling that doesn't hang around, because they know how to deal with it in a constructive way.

Those of us whose MI is more rocky have usually had to deal with what I call 'road blocks' on their learning life-path. Here are some that you may recognise.

Common 'road-blocks' on the development path to MI

1. What can stop us from having the mental ability to ***distinguish right from wrong****?*

- Being too young: our brain's cognitive abilities develop gradually and at a different pace in each individual child.
- Having brain damage or deficiency: this can be present when someone is born, or it can happen at any time during our lives. We are just at the start of being able to find and diagnose many of these problems.
- Suffering from a mental illness: which, when it is active, can sometimes affect our powers of reasoning (e.g. depression, OCD, PSTD, bipolar, schizophrenia or dementia).
- Being stressed: when our brain is overloaded and too tired we may not reason so efficiently. Our default responses,

which are neurologically 'set' in our brains, can take over from our reasoning. Many of these were developed in our childhood, but we now know that frequently repeated responses and traumatic experiences in adulthood can also affect the kind of auto-emotional responses we experience.

*2. What can stop us from straying away from **universal principles**?*

- Not knowing what they are: many children nowadays grow up without receiving sufficient moral knowledge and guidance. For many centuries religion was the main channel through which these universal principles were taught and enforced. Parents would further reinforce this learning by discipline and role-modelling at home. Nowadays much of our world has become secularised and the responsibility for this 'teaching' role is not so clearly defined.
- When one or more of these principles clash with our needs – for example, someone who is hungry or has a child who is sick might put their need for help before the principle of compassion for someone who is even needier.
- A culture clash – although these principles are in theory universal, every country and every culture within it may differ in how much they want to abide by these principles. For example, when an older person gets onto a crowded train, in some countries a younger person will immediately offer them a seat. In others, where respect for elders is not an accepted principle, they will not.
- Prejudice – the acquired belief that some humans are of lesser value than others can override almost all the universal principles in one fell swoop.

*3. What can stop us from keeping our **values and goals** in line with universal principles?*

- Adopting an overly *laissez-faire* attitude to our life – the majority of my new clients struggle to name the values and the goals which they use or would like to use to guide their choices and plans. They have drifted through life bumping into opportunities and people who pull and push them in all manner of directions.

- Caring more about either our goals or our personal values than the universal principles.
- Personality traits such as arrogance, passiveness and courage.

*4. What can stop us from dealing well with **moral dilemmas and competing desires**?*

- Being spoilt as a child – or even as an adult! Being given almost anything we wanted.
- Never getting the practice of dealing with dilemmas because others, such as parents, bosses and paternalistic politicians, make all the decisions.
- Preferring the peace of 'giving up' rather than going through the torture of having to decide.

*5. What can stop us from having **the motivation and will power** to keep in line with universal principles?*

- Not having good enough assertiveness skills to be able to stand up for what is right.
- Believing that our opinion isn't as valuable as those who are not respecting the principles.
- Fear of being bullied or ridiculed because we are too 'goody-goody'.
- Being too tired and/or too dejected to care.

As you read the above, other examples and ideas on the subject may have come to mind. My examples as to why the foundations of someone's MI might not be very firm are certainly not exhaustive. The following exercise will help you to clarify what might have hindered you in the development of your own MI and what you could do to correct that influence.

EXERCISE: DEALING WITH MY OWN PERSONAL 'ROAD-BLOCKS' TO ACHIEVING GOOD ENOUGH MORAL INTELLIGENCE

1. Re-read the above section and note down the 'road-blocks' that chime with your experiences.
2. Beside each one, write down some action you could take if you spot this happening again. For example, in response to road-block number 1: *Do regular relaxation exercises*; or for number 5: *Keep my self-esteem boosted and learn assertiveness.*

Even if you normally have very good MI, there are times when all of us go through rocky patches. After all, in our everyday contemporary lives our morality is being constantly pulled and pushed in different directions, many of which we have already looked at in Chapter 2 such as:

- competing political and religious philosophies;
- contradictory ideas about what constitutes a 'good' parent, teacher, banker, charity worker, etc.;
- conflicting ideas about how to spend our money, dress ourselves, dispose of rubbish or drive a car in order to become a 'decent' citizen.

In addition, as individuals we all at some time or other encounter difficulties when a decision confronts us with our own competing values. For example:

At work:

- Should I: become a doctor or a banker/start my own business or stay in this boring job which is secure/make four of the young new recruits redundant or three experienced managers who all have families/work or stay at home while the children are young?

Over finance:

- Should I: buy a house that we can only afford if we both work shifts/send the kids to private schools now we can afford to do so/get a new sofa when the old one is still okay and loads of people haven't even got a home/get him an iPad on credit just because most of his classmates have one?

In relationships:

- Should I: tell him I have had an affair even though it's now over/get a divorce or stick it out for the kids for the next 15 years/give Mum more time even if John kicks off about us never having time together/just tell Dad he is going into a home when I think he will hate it/spend more time with fun friends and give up the ones who are so needy/tell her what I know about his past or let her enjoy the relationship while it lasts?

An apparently constant stream of these kinds of dilemmas makes many people resigned to life-long guilt. I can't promise that the following exercises will render you totally guilt-free, but they will minimise the burden considerably. They certainly have for me.

Guilt, as we know, is a value judgement. We need to be able to assess as rapidly as possible whether it is truly our value judgement or whether it originates from elsewhere. Knowing and prioritising our own personal values is therefore crucial. I have designed this next exercise as a foundation step for enabling you to do this. It is not one that you will be able to do very quickly, but it is worth doing well, as it is crucial for managing your guilt.

EXERCISE: CLARIFYING YOUR PERSONAL VALUES

Here is a long list of values, qualities and traits. Obviously some are going to leap off the page as being very important to you. Others will make you wonder why they have been included. We are all so wonderfully different!

Achievement
Adventurousness
Altruism
Ambition
Balance
Being the best
Belonging
Calmness
Carefulness
Challenge
Cheerfulness
Clear-mindedness
Commitment
Community
Compassion
Competitiveness
Contentment
Control
Cooperation
Correctness
Courageousness
Courtesy
Creativity
Curiosity
Decisiveness
Democracy
Dependability
Determination
Diligence
Discipline
Discretion
Diversity
Economy
Effectiveness
Efficiency
Elegance
Empathy
Enjoyment
Enthusiasm
Equality
Excellence
Excitement
Expertise
Expressiveness
Fairness
Faith
Family
Fidelity
Focus
Freedom
Fun
Generosity
Goodness
Growth
Happiness
Health
Helping others
Honesty
Honour
Humility
Independence
Ingenuity
Inner peace
Insightfulness
Intelligence
Intuition
Joy
Justice
Leadership
Legacy
Love
Loyalty
Making a difference
Merit
Obedience
Openness
Order

Originality	Self-fulfilment	Structure
Patriotism	Self-control	Success
Peace	Selflessness	Support
Perfection	Self-reliance	Teamwork
Positivity	Sensitivity	Thoughtfulness
Practicality	Serenity	Tolerance
Preparedness	Service	Tradition
Professionalism	Shrewdness	Trustworthiness
Prudence	Simplicity	Truth-seeking
Quality	Soundness	Understanding
Reliability	Speed	Uniqueness
Resourcefulness	Spontaneity	Usefulness
Restraint	Stability	Vitality
Security	Strength	

Action:

- Note down (or mark) six values in relation to each of these ten questions:

1. Which would make you feel most good about yourself?
2. Which would you be most proud to receive a compliment on at work?
3. Which would you most want a partner in your personal life to value you for?
4. Which would you most like to overhear your neighbours praising you for?
5. Which would you like to see a grown-up child of yours mention in a thank-you card to you?
6. Which would your Mum (or a key mother figure) have felt most proud to hear said about you?
7. Which would your Dad (or a key father figure) have felt most proud to hear said about you?
8. Which one would you like one of your best friends to say they appreciated in you?
9. Which one would you like a different kind of friend to say they appreciate about you?
10. Which would you like to hear mentioned, should you ever receive a life-time service award from your country?

- Review your answers and tick the values that you see in another answer (some may have more than one tick).
- Make a list of the ticked values, putting the ones that have the most ticks at the top.
- Make a final **hierarchical list of ten of these values**, putting the most important at the top and the least important last.
- Over the next two weeks take this list around with you. Read and reflect on it regularly. Notice which of these values you are respecting in your everyday life, and those that you are finding difficult to live by. If possible, talk to friends about your list and note their comments.
- At the end of the fortnight (the date should be noted in your diary!), review your list and alter the order of the values if you need to do so. You can also replace some of the values with others on my list or with others that you would prefer to include. You can update this list as many times as you wish during your life. Your values usually do change as your life develops.
- Consult this list whenever you feel guilty and notice which of your values you have not been respecting. Make a resolution to do something immediately to repair this situation. Remember to reward yourself with a treat when you have done so.
- Also, consult this list whenever you feel stuck with a moral dilemma. It will help you to be more decisive. All moral dilemmas deserve quality time so they can be carefully thought through, but do set a time limit for doing this, otherwise you may not make the decision until it is too late – and just think how guilty you would feel then!

Personal life rules

The next exercise will help you to apply the work you have hopefully just done in everyday life. I created it many years ago after being asked this question by a journalist: *'What are your three top rules for leading a happy life?'* I responded spontaneously, as journalists rarely ever give you time to think.

1. Be true to yourself and your values.
2. See the positive in change, however unwelcome it may seem.
3. Spend more time than you think you can afford on the relationships that matter most to you.

Over the next few months I found that I was frequently referring to these rules and finding them quite challenging. I realised that each rule reflected an issue over which I had truly struggled.

- Firstly, I was a people pleaser, so I lived largely by others' values. I didn't even know what my own were.
- Secondly, I was a negative thinker, mainly because my life up to that point had 'proved' to me that change was bad news.
- Thirdly, I was very cynical about relationships and rarely let anyone get close to me. Close relationships had, for the most part, brought me more pain than joy.

Nowadays, I rarely have any trouble living by my first life rule. However, the other two can still sometimes be tough to respect. For example, on the two occasions when my husband has been made redundant, my auto-response was to feel fearful and depressed. This happened in spite of our many joint years of professional experience in the field. Over and over again I had witnessed how redundancy can become very good news. My negative belief was so deeply embedded in my mind as a child that it comes on immediately when I am stressed. My number-two rule, however, will now kick in and help me get back to my adult self.

With regard to my number-three rule, as my diary rarely has a blank day I almost always feel too busy to fit in an unexpected opportunity to catch up with friends who may be passing through London. As I am about to say, *'What a pity,'* my number-three rule prods me. It has been an invaluable tool in helping me to reprioritise time for these opportunities.

Many of my clients have found the following exercise helpful. I hope you do, too. It should certainly help diminish your guilt.

EXERCISE: MY THREE PERSONAL LIFE RULES

- Think of three old habits that stop you from keeping in line with the values you want to live by today. These are probably going to be among the values you marked from the list in the last exercise.
- Create three life rules for yourself that will help you to check these habits. Write them out and place them in a prominent place where you will encounter them regularly. Read them out loud from time to time to fix them in your brain.
- Show them to friends who could remind you of them when they see you slipping back into your old ways.
- Change your rules when they become redundant and create new ones if you still are not living well enough by your own values. (Guilt will send you the alert!)

With integrity, you have nothing to fear, since you have nothing to hide. With integrity, you will do the right thing, so you will have no guilt.

ZIG ZIGLAR, HIGHLY SUCCESSFUL BUSINESSMAN AND MOTIVATIONAL COACH

Skill 2: Rational thinking

What really frightens and dismays us is not external events themselves, but the way in which we think about them. It is not things that disturb us, but our interpretation of their significance.

EPICTETUS, GREEK PHILOSOPHER

Isn't it amazing that a Greek philosopher who lived nearly two millennia ago was making people aware of how much their thinking could cause emotional disturbance and a negative outcome? Unfortunately, too many of us haven't quite kicked our bad-thinking habits and still need some help.

The ability to think rationally is, as I have already mentioned, crucial for both feeling guilt and managing it well. Firstly, we need to be able to distinguish between guilt that is justified and that which is not. Secondly, if we are truly guilty, we need to rationally assess the best way to make effective amends. Thirdly, if our guilt responses have been faulty we need to examine and learn from them.

A particular form of therapy called Cognitive Behavioural Therapy (CBT) has recently become very popular. Its aim is to help people who have developed mental-health problems due to negative thinking based on irrational beliefs. Many of its ideas developed from the work of a psychologist called Albert Ellis who from the 1960s to the 1990s developed what is known as Rational Emotive Behaviour Therapy (REBT). My examples and suggestions in this section have been based partly on ideas I have adapted from both CBT and REBT, as well as strategies that I have developed in my own practice.

> **Rational beliefs bring us closer to getting good results in the real world.**
>
> ALBERT ELLIS, FOUNDER OF RATIONAL EMOTIVE BEHAVIOUR THERAPY

I have selected the three following strategies because they work well with guilt. Try out each of them and use the ones that work best for you. Please also do the exercises so that you can see how they might be used in situations where you feel guilty. This will make the strategy more meaningful and memorable.

Reframing

What rational-thinking skills help us to do is become more aware of the links between our feelings, thoughts and behaviour and the consequences. When we start thinking negatively, we need to first analyse the problem by looking at these links. Our next step is to 'reframe' our thoughts to bring them in line with positive rational thinking. My examples will show how that can (and usually does) affect our behaviour and its consequences.

Situation 1: Grace has just realised she's given in to her child again when she didn't want to.

Feelings: Guilt and hopelessness.

> **Thoughts**: I am a useless parent; my kids are going to grow up spoilt and arrogant.

> **Behaviour:** Asks her husband to deal with these situations.

> **Consequences:** Her children and her husband lose some of their respect for her. Grace's self-esteem plummets.

The reframe:

Feelings: Guilt and hopelessness.

> **Thoughts:** I love my children but I do need to de-stress and learn to be more assertive with them.

> **Behaviour:** Buys a book on assertiveness. Asks her husband to help her practise the skills she needs.

> **Consequences:** Grace does learn how to say no to her children when she chooses to do so. Her self-confidence is boosted and she does not feel guilty.

Situation 2: Sean has just made a misjudgement when overtaking a car.

Feelings: Guilt and shock.

> **Thoughts**: I could have killed myself and others. How thoughtless and stupid! What if I'd had Anne with me? What an idiot I am.

> **Behaviour**: He crawls along in the slow lane for the rest of the journey.

> **Consequences**: Sean is late for work and feels even more guilt and suffers with poor concentration all day.

The reframe:

Feelings: Guilt and shock.

> **Thoughts**: That was too close a call. It was a dreadful mistake to make. I guess I was too stressed about being late for work. I need to chill out.

> **Behaviour**: Sean stopped as soon as he could. He did some deep breathing and stretches and had a drink of water. He texted his boss to say that he would be a few minutes late as he had an incident on the motorway.

> **Consequences:** Sean did some more stretches and deep breathing before going in to work. He 'confessed' to his boss what he had done. He said he would take a shorter lunch break to make up the time lost, and that he had decided from now on to leave for work 15 minutes earlier than he had been doing. He is satisfied that he has learned an important lesson and has no residual guilt.

EXERCISE: REFRAMING MY THINKING WHEN I FEEL GUILTY

- Recall one mistake. Note down the negative feelings, thoughts, behaviour and consequences that occurred (or could have occurred). Reframe each of these in the way I have done with the examples above.
- Think of one personality failing you have (e.g. being late, eating junk food, not suffering fools gladly). Note down your negative reactions (or possible negative reactions) to this trait and the consequences. Reframe each as above.

Background beliefs checklist

Albert Ellis, the psychologist I mentioned earlier, identified 12 common irrational beliefs that people who habitually think negatively tend to hold. I have found that a number of them are usually lurking in the minds of people who are troubled with guilt. The following exercise will help you identify the ones that may be hindering you from dealing rationally with your guilt.

EXERCISE: BACKGROUND BELIEFS CHECKLIST

Albert Ellis's 12 common irrational beliefs

☐ 1. It is a dire necessity for adults to be loved by significant others for almost everything they do.

☐ 2. Certain acts are awful or wicked, and people who perform such acts should be severely damned.

☐ 3. It is horrible when things are not the way we like them to be.

☐ 4. Human misery is invariably externally caused and is forced on us by outside people and events.

☐ 5. If something is or may be dangerous or fearsome, we should be terribly upset and endlessly obsess about it.

☐ 6. It is easier to avoid than to face life difficulties and self-responsibilities.

☐ 7. We absolutely need something other or stronger or greater than ourselves on which to rely.

☐ 8. We should be thoroughly competent, intelligent and achieving in all possible respects.

☐ 9. Because something once strongly affected our life, it should indefinitely affect it.

☐ 10. We must have certain and perfect control over things.

☐ 11. Human happiness can be achieved by inertia and inaction.

☐ 12. We have virtually no control over our emotions and we cannot help feeling disturbed about things.

• • •

- Tick the beliefs that you think may be lodged in your mind. Add, in your own words, any of your own that come to mind.
- Rewrite the irrational beliefs that are relevant to your reaction in a situation. Rewrite them so that they form a personal rational statement. For example, No. 10: *I can never be certain that I have complete control, but I can do my level best to make sure that things will work out well.*
- Use this list as a checklist when you are stuck in a guilt trap. Transform the ones that are relevant to your situation into positive rational statements.

The GEE strategy

This is a simple strategy, which I devised and have successfully used for very many years to help with guilt. It is easy to remember and can be done very quickly. It focuses on the three most common bad-thinking habits that negative thinkers tend to have.

1. Generalising from one particular mistake or failure.
2. Exaggerating the impact.
3. Excluding any positive options for action.

It is an ideal strategy to use as soon as your guilt has been triggered. You can teach it to your nearest and dearest, too! Ask them to say *'GEE!'* as soon as they hear you slipping into one or more of these habits. They can even do that quietly when you are out with others, as no one will know what it means.

Here are some examples of it being used with different kinds of guilt.

GENERALISING

Survivor guilt is incurable. I have known three people who were Holocaust survivors who committed suicide with it. And it has ruined the lives of many tsunami survivors. You can't remove experiences like that from your mind.

> *Survivor guilt is hard to deal with. But there are more people who have been able to move on positively with their lives than those who haven't. I don't need to forget those who were lost. I can find uplifting and comforting rituals to help me commemorate them regularly. I have a choice whether to remain defeated by this guilt or not.*

Exaggerating

Of course I feel bad about what I did! But she never listens to me so there's absolutely no point in apologising or trying to put it right. I've got to get away. We will kill each other otherwise.

> *She's your mother. She has been listening to you all your life. You have fallen out many times and found a way to just agree to differ. You love each other so there is a point in trying to talk to her again. One day you will be in a position to live independently and it will be easier.*

Excluding

The only way to rid myself of the guilt I feel for being as well paid as I am is to sell up everything, give it to the poor and live like Gandhi.

> *The truth is that there are many other options open to you. You could take a sabbatical to work with a charity. Or you could use some of your wealth and skills to create or support not-for-profit initiatives, or become more politically active. Any of these and other options could help millions of people to have a better lifestyle.*

EXERCISE: THE GEE STRATEGY

- Think of a mistake you have made or a failure that did trigger justified guilt in you. Write down what negative thoughts you had in response. Use the GEE strategy to assess the rationality of your thinking.
- Think of a guilt preoccupation that you have fairly regularly, e.g. *I am a bad parent because I work too much; I am unfair to my staff because I am an incorrigible perfectionist; I am my own worst enemy – that's why all my relationships break down.*

- Write down some of the accusatory self-talk you might use when you have these kinds of guilty thoughts. Use the GEE strategy again to check out the rationality of your thinking.

Finally, here's another simple quick fix derived from Cognitive Behavioural Therapy training. It is also easy to remember and use, but it does require you to have first clarified your own true values and know your own bad-thinking habits. The exercises on values in my section on moral intelligence (see pages 76–78) should have helped you already in this respect.

The Three Cs quick fix

Catch it

Once you (or a close friend) have spotted one of your regular negative thoughts, imagine yourself catching it in the air as it enters your head.

Example: *Mum was right. I should have stuck it out for my son's sake and not got divorced.*

Check it

Ask yourself:

- Is it rational? *Not necessarily; only partly.*
- Is there any evidence for it? *The research findings often conflict.*
- Is this what I would say to a good friend? *No, certainly not.*
- Do I need to seek the opinion of others? *No, I thought about it very carefully before I made the decision. I chose what I thought was the lesser of the two evils for all of us.*

Change it

Substitute the negative thought for a new positive one:

> *I made what I believed was the best decision and I am doing my very best to minimise the hurtful impact on Tom.*

The best years of your life are the ones in which you decide your problems are your own. You do not blame them on your mother, the ecology or the president. You realise that you control your own destiny.

ALBERT ELLIS, FOUNDER OF RATIONAL EMOTIVE BEHAVIOUR THERAPY

If your negative thinking persists then it would be a good idea to see a doctor. It could be that you have become depressed and need some extra help. Your doctor may advise some medication or refer you to a counsellor or a therapist. If you have to wait a while, keep trying these exercises and doing plenty of fun activities.

Skill 3: Confident communication

Guilt, whether it is rational or not, tends to make us adopt a more passive or aggressive style of communication than we might otherwise use. This is true even for people who are normally confident and communicate well. We are rarely consciously aware of this effect. So if guilt is around, it is well worth taking a little time to prepare before you speak, text, type or write.

Firstly, we must remember that there are two kinds of confidence: inner and outer. To achieve confident communication we need both. Inwardly, our self-esteem must be high; we must have enough self-knowledge to know our communication strengths and weaknesses; we must be sure of what we can achieve, and we must feel positive enough to believe that our communication can be effective.

To appear externally confident we must have the skills to communicate effectively, a physical presence that attracts attention (but doesn't shout for it), assertiveness skills to protect ourselves and stand up for our beliefs and needs, and emotional control to ensure that our feelings don't sabotage our efforts to communicate our message.

To achieve this level of super-confidence is of course a challenge for anyone. But when you are feeling guilty, it can seem impossible. For the moment, let's aim once again for a 'good enough' standard. To make this relatively easy for you, here are some strategies that will get you started.

The Three Ps for confident communication when you are feeling guilty

1. **Postponement**. While you are feeling guilty, try to never seize an opportunity to confess, apologise or discuss the situation before you have had time to properly think it through and prepare yourself. Should somebody attempt to start discussing it either face-to-face or on the phone or by text or email, respond positively: *'Yes, I certainly would like to talk to you about it but ...'/'I am pleased you rang but ...'* If you need to use a white lie to justify the postponement, use one of the classic stallers confident communicators use, such as: *'I'm just about to go into a meeting right now'* (the business person's favourite!)/*'I'm in the middle of cooking.'/'You've caught me on a madly busy day.'/ 'I haven't got the information in front of me now'* (the politician's favourite!). Then suggest a few times when you could get back to them. Be careful to give yourself enough time to prepare (to avoid what guilt might prompt you to say, such as, *'When would be convenient for you?'*).

2. **Preparation**: When we are feeling guilty we are rarely as articulate as we need to be. You should prepare by thinking through what you want to say. Writing helps to engage the cognitive centre of your brain quickly, which is why I recommend always having a small notebook or tablet handy. You can use it to compose a quick script to explain what happened or to make a good apology. If the situation is very important, or your guilt feels complex, I would strongly recommend that you try using one of the strategies in this book to guide you. To analyse the situation and clarify your share of the responsibility, use my new strategy, the DREAM Repair Kit in Chapter 5. If you want to make an apology, follow the guidelines below.

3. **Practice**: Ideally, it helps to do this with someone else. It makes it more real and they can also give you feedback. If you are on your own, stand in front of a long mirror to practise saying your script. But before you do, you must rid your body of tension. Do some relaxation stretches (neck and face) and diaphragmatic breathing. Stand or sit, well balanced, with both feet on the ground. Release any crossed or curled limbs and ensure your stance is upright. Eye contact should not be the staring kind, but looking directly into the other person's eyes at least 50 per cent of the time. Don't be afraid of pausing or checking your notes.

How to make a confident apology

The manner in which you apologise undoubtedly affects the outcome. Unfortunately guilt tends to make us either over-apologise in an annoyingly 'wimpish' way, or make us defensive, when our apologies can come across as half-hearted or even glib. An apology delivered confidently is much more likely to be believed and readily accepted. I have devised an outline for a script that I hope will be a useful guide. Those of you who are familiar with some of my other books will know that scripting is one of my favourite strategies. This one is similar to others that I have used, but has some key adaptations for use when making apologies.

Scripting is not intended to be the only answer to problems; it is simply a way to start the problem-solving process in a confident and positive way. Because of the way the script is written, edited and rehearsed, it will be listened to more attentively. It engages the listener because it is concise and considerate of their feelings, and concerned with finding a good, realistic outcome for both parties. Of course, the timing should be right. If the person concerned is still too shocked, hurt or angry, you cannot expect your apology to be accepted. You may have to return again and repeat it later. If they won't see you at first, you can use the script outline to compose a letter or an email. Then, later, you could use it to suggest ways that you could make amends.

First, I will outline the four steps of the script and give you some relevant dos and don'ts in each section to bear in mind. Then, I will give you some real-life examples to show you how it can be applied.

As you know I am British and my examples are therefore going to reflect my culture. If you are living or working in a different culture, you may have to adapt your style a little. The basics will be the same, but the verbal and non-verbal language may need some modifying. What is considered confident in one culture may be interpreted as aggressive or even passive in another. So do try to check out any scripts that you write with someone who is known to be confident and assertive within your cultural environment.

There are four stages to prepare:

1. **S**ummary
2. **E**motion
3. **A**pology and/or **A**mends
4. **P**ay-off

Use this mnemonic to prompt you to remember the first letter of each.

Script **E**very **A**pology **P**ositively

EXAMPLE A: DEREK'S CHRISTMAS DILEMMA

Derek's parents live in the North of the UK – a five- or six-hour drive away from his home in London. His father had recently had an operation and his mother asked him to ask his wife, Wanda, if the family could come to their house for Christmas, as his father's spirits were very low. The original plan was to go to Wanda's parents' in Poland that year.

Derek needed to ring his mother to tell her that the family was still going ahead with the trip to his in-laws. Wanda had said that the tickets were not exchangeable and her parents had already arranged too many activities for the children for her to ask them to cancel. Derek had also recently been told that he had to go to the US for a week in early December for work, so he would not be able to visit them until late January.

He was very anxious about making the call, afraid that his mother might start crying. As you can imagine, he was feeling very guilty about not giving his parents the support they needed. He put off ringing them for two weeks because '*I just didn't know how to tell them.*' He nearly decided he would have to write a letter, even though he knew that would upset them even more. Then Wanda remembered being told by a friend about scripting, and together they wrote and rehearsed this script to start off the phone call.

Derek's script for a phone call to his mother:

Hi, Mum, you remember that a couple of weeks ago we discussed the possibility of us changing our Christmas arrangements. I'm afraid this isn't going to be possible. And unfortunately I now have a work commitment in the US in December, so I cannot even pop up to see you before Christmas. [**S**ummary.]

I guess you and Dad will be very disappointed and may feel unsupported by me [expressing empathic **E**motion]. I feel very bad, too, about not being able to be with you at Christmas [Derek's emotion].

I hope you will accept my way of trying to make up for this. I am buying you a tablet and I have arranged with Janet [Derek's sister] to bring it to you on Boxing Day so we can all have a video conversation. I will come up some time in January and teach you more about how you can use it. [**A**pology and **A**mends.]

It is so easy to use that you and Dad will be able to call the kids and us regularly, and you will be able to call Janet on it as well. I'm sure this will help us to all feel much closer and will cheer Dad up, too. He is going to love some of the word games and will be able to watch football any time he chooses. [A win/win **P**ositive pay-off.]

Derek's mother didn't cry. Indeed, she said she understood. They now have regular video chats and plan to spend Easter together.

EXAMPLE B: PROJECT LEADER BOB'S FAILURE TO DEAL WITH A STAFF CONFLICT

Bob's team have for months been moaning to each other about one of their colleagues, Brian. Although no one complained formally to Bob, he knew about this but chose to ignore it. (Conflict resolution was not one of his strengths.)

Eventually, Brian behaved so rudely to the deputy leader of the project, Linda, that she decided to resign.

After investigating the incident, Bob knew that he had to take disciplinary action. He gave Brian a formal warning. On receiving this, Brian was very angry and extremely insulting to Bob. He also handed in his resignation, which Bob accepted. He was very nervous about discussing this incident at the team's next meeting. They were all aware that Linda had quickly secured a position with a competitor, so there was no hope of her returning.

Bob knew he was guilty of avoiding this staff issue, which had then become a serious crisis for his team. Now he wanted to apologise to the team, ask for their support and re-motivate them. This was his script.

Bob's script to open his next staff meeting

As we all know, the problem with Brian's disruptive behaviour has been going on for some months. I am well aware that if I had taken action earlier we would not have lost Linda at this crucial time. [**S**ummary.]

I know that some of you are angry with me, and I am guessing that others of you, at the very least, feel let down by me. I do understand why you would feel this way and I do feel regret at not having dealt with the situation earlier. [Empathy with their **E**motion and expressing his emotion of regret.]

I want to apologise to you all and assure you that it will not happen again. This has been a wake-up call for me. I have already started executive coaching sessions to help me improve my managerial skills. I would very much appreciate your honest feedback about how I am doing over the next few months. I promise that I will make every effort to replace Linda as soon as possible. In the meantime I will work overtime to ensure that I can cover her responsibilities. [**A**pology and **A**mends.]

I am confident that we will soon get back to working together as the excellent team we undoubtedly are, and I know that the project will be a great success. [A win/win **P**ositive pay-off.]

If you would like more help with confident communication, I have written extensively on the subject in other books (take a look at *Super Confidence* and *Assert Yourself*). There are also many courses available on the subject. I think you will find that many of the other techniques, exercises and tips in this book will also firm up your skills in this important area.

Skill 4: Emotional management

When any difficult emotion, such as guilt, is triggered, the chances are that our physiological stress mode has also switched on. This is particularly true if two of guilt's buddies – fear and anger – have also been added to the emotional brew.

Emotional management is a very big topic and can be perhaps the biggest challenge for anyone concerned with self-improvement. It is only recently that people have taken the subject seriously. Before then people thought they were at the mercy of their feelings. Most of us grew up hearing adults say: *'I can't help feeling this way'; I know she's bad for me, but I can't help loving her'; 'I didn't mean to shout at him, my irritation just burst out'; 'I was shaking with fear, I couldn't stop myself'; 'I know it doesn't make sense but I can't help feeling guilty'; 'You made me so angry saying what you did that I couldn't stop myself from throwing it'.*

> **Logic will not change an emotion, but action will.**
>
> ANONYMOUS

We may have been told we were '*stupid*' to feel so and so, or that we '*shouldn't*' feel this or that, and we should feel something different. But nobody told us how we could start or stop feeling our emotions. I think this is partly because our emotions feel so much part of the fabric of ourselves that it is quite threatening to talk about the subject. It was certainly like that for me. It wasn't until I reached my ultimate point when my feelings became a threat to my life and my children's welfare that I tentatively tried out some emotional management strategies. Even then, I think I could only do so under the guise of becoming more assertive. I justified my attendance at courses by saying that I would be able to 'fight' more effectively for my children's needs and those of my underprivileged and sick clients. Most people I now train today do this as well. Many, indeed, have to get a better grip on their feelings – their employers have threatened their jobs or the courts have threatened alternative 'punishments'.

These attitudes may now seem old-fashioned, but they are still lurking around in our subconscious minds. You may find yourself resisting the emotional management strategies. You could start by dismissing them as too simplistic. If you do, tell yourself that the simpler they are, the more likely they are to work (this is true!). The parts of our brain that we are trying to get more under our control are very primitive.

Another 'resistance' line to watch out for sounds something like this: *'I don't want to become a programmed robot ... I like being a sensitive and passionate person.'*

The answer to this argument is that people who know how to control their feelings are much freer to be sensitive and passionate. This is because they are confident in their ability to recover from any inconvenience, disappointment or hurt that their deep feelings may bring.

The physiological process of the stress response

The stress response is a process that takes place within our bodies when our brain 'notices' what it considers to be a threat to us. It is usually switched on when we are feeling a difficult emotion such as guilt, anxiety, fear or anger. We may or may not notice that changes have taken place in our bodies.

The stress response's function is to prepare us to either fight or quickly take flight. It is commonly called the fight or flight response. Nowadays, a third kind of response has been identified and is often added in the description: freeze. This is doing nothing. It includes what psychologists call denial. You behave as though there is no stressful threat, even though the physiological stress response is operating. It is actually a common response in our contemporary human world and very relevant to our management of guilt.

The stress response was designed for our primitive ancestors, who were facing physical threats. This is what happens:

- Certain hormones are stimulated, which engage the sympathetic branch of our autonomic nervous system.
- Our eyes dilate to improve our vision.
- Our heart rate increases to circulate blood more quickly to vital organs and our respiration increases to provide increased oxygen to the rapidly circulating blood.
- The muscles in our arms and legs tense up to enable us to move quickly and precisely.
- Our breathing changes. Instead of breathing slowly and gently from our lower lungs, we begin to breathe rapidly and shallowly from our upper lungs. This shift not only increases the amount of oxygen in our bloodstream, but it also quickly 'blows off' an increasing amount of carbon dioxide. In a physical emergency we are producing excess carbon dioxide, so this breathing rate is essential.

The effect on our mind is that our thinking speed shoots up so we can quickly decide whether to fight, take flight or freeze.

In humans and in many animals when difficult feelings are also involved, the amygdala centre in the brain is activated. This is also a primitive response centre, which is linked to our emotional system. Neurological science is developing fast and may soon give us more insight into how the amygdala works. My current understanding is that at least one of its functions is to create blueprints, which are basically ready-made strategies for dealing with emotionally charged emergencies. These are derived from the amygdala's 'impression' of which strategies have worked well for both our ancestors and us in the past. So they are created both from our nature (our genes) and our nurture (our life experiences, particularly in childhood and during traumatic times as an adult).

In theory that all sounds good, but in practice it doesn't work too well for most of our needs today. Our modern crises require much more carefully thought through responses, rather than these crude blueprints. Unlike our forefathers, we've now developed more sophisticated centres in our brain to deal with stressors. The problem is that people don't always use these cognitive abilities to think thoroughly through their options. Indeed, many mental-health crises occur <u>because</u> people are still responding to problems in both our external and internal worlds with their primitive stress response.

The effect of this 'misuse' of the stress response is that people over-react to minor issues or under-react to more serious threats. The amygdala's blueprints may have worked well for us as children, and still do in times of war or major traumas, but may not go down so well with our boss, or our nearest and dearest. Indeed, these past-their-sell-by-date strategies can actually often be counterproductive, as Terry's story illustrates:

Terry had a father who would lose his temper in a frightening way whenever his son did anything naughty. His mother never stepped in to defend him and, indeed, threatened to tell his father if he did anything he shouldn't. So when Terry's ball broke a glass pane in the neighbour's garden, he was too frightened to tell his parents. As nobody appeared to notice the broken pane, there were no repercussions. Terry, however, became very secretive from then on about all his misdemeanours. Most of the time his strategy was very successful and it became a blueprint stress response, which came on whenever he did something that made him feel guilty.

As an adult, Terry's habitual method of handling guilt caused him tension headaches and self-esteem issues, but it didn't get him into any big trouble for many years. One day, however, he damaged another car while parking in the underground car park at work. No one else seemed to be around. So, as usual, Terry felt guilty, but he did nothing about it.

As it happened, the damaged car belonged to the new Head of Finance. This man found a small trace of paint on his car. He knew it belonged to Terry's car because it was the only one in the garage that was the same colour. Terry hadn't noticed the paint in the darkness of the car park.

The next day the Head of Finance circulated the registration number to all the departmental heads, asking if anyone knew who owned the offending car. Terry's boss was told whose car it was. He confronted Terry, who denied doing the damage. But, as it happened, his boss was an ex-police officer and was well trained in spotting non-verbal signs of guilt. He persisted with his questioning, and eventually Terry confessed.

Terry didn't lose his job, but he was not given the promotion he thought he was due. When he started applying for other jobs and didn't get them, he guessed that his boss was not giving him good references. He couldn't prove this as the references must have been given by phone or face-to-face. (Terry's world of work was a niche and small one.)

Terry learned an important lesson about guilt management, but paid a very heavy price in the process.

Guilt's best feeling friends are fear, anger and shame, so these are the ones we will address. Our goal will be to tame these. We can't, and don't want to, eradicate any of them because they can all serve useful functions. But when they are 'playing together' in response to guilt, they can become severely troublesome. We can wind up with a mixed bag of confusing emotion inside us that is difficult to control, as this story about Ken illustrates.

Ken has a secret gambling addiction. He **feels guilty** about the vast debts he has accrued. He is **terrified** that if he confides in his wife she will leave him and take his daughter. He has nightmares every night.

He goes to see a GP and is refused sleeping tablets. He **loses his temper** with the doctor and shouts abuse at her. The receptionist enters and asks if she should call for help. Ken feels extremely **ashamed**. He apologises and leaves the surgery.

Ken, instead of returning home, goes to a nearby pub and tries to drown his cauldron of feelings. The first drink doesn't work. So he drinks some more, and then more. He starts arguing with another man in the pub and being threatening towards him. Predictably, Ken ends up at the police station and receives a warning. His wife is called and asked to collect him.

Ken's story is quite dramatic and depressing, but it does illustrate how these emotions of fear, anger and shame often work in conjunction with guilt. These emotions can similarly be linked even when our guilt might be irrational or very minimal. A more everyday example might be a parent who is so preoccupied with their guilt about not being a good-enough parent that they start to become irritable with their spouse and fearfully overprotective of their children.

And this 'emotional partnership' can, of course, work the other way round. For example, someone snaps at a new junior at work and on the way home starts feeling guilty. They become so anxious about repeating their unprovoked irritable behaviour that they become uncomfortably patronising to all junior staff and don't give them the negative feedback they need.

> **Stress is not what happens to us. It's our response TO what happens. And RESPONSE is something we can choose.**
>
> MAUREEN KILLORAN, AMERICAN LIFE COACH

In this short section, I cannot deal in any depth with management of all the difficult emotions related to guilt, so I have chosen to focus on dealing with the stress response and a few simple strategies to help you control your fear and anger. There is also one for shameful guilt on page 171.

Three quick fixes for turning off your stress response

The sooner you learn and practise these quick fixes the better. Don't put off doing this until you feel the tension and other uncomfortable feelings of the stress response. It will be almost impossible to learn a new technique then. If you develop the habit of using at least one of them daily, this will keep you in good mental and physical shape and more able to face any challenge that should come your way. They all ensure that your heart and brain are working as efficiently as they are able.

STRETCH, SQUEEZE AND BREATHE

Wherever you are, if you start to feel guilty, use this exercise to calm your pulse rate. It will only take two to three minutes.

Squeeze and release at least one set of muscles three times. If you are sitting at a table in a restaurant or in a meeting at work, you can also use your calves, thighs and hands without anyone noticing. Even if you can only use your toes, that will help. Cover your mouth with one hand (as people often do when they are listening attentively). Then you can take a couple of deep breaths down into the bottom of your stomach without anyone noticing. Breathe out very slowly each time. With your hand over your face, no one will notice you have pursed your lips to ensure your breath comes out slowly.

If you can go somewhere where no one can see you (such as the loo!), pull some very peculiar faces. Stretch your facial muscles almost to their limits. Hold for a second or two, and then slowly release them. Finally, do as many stretches and squeezes of other muscles as your space and time will allow.

MAGIC MENTAL REVIVER

This technique can be used literally anywhere, such as sitting in a waiting area or a car park. It will work even better if you can find somewhere to lie down or sit. It will not only switch off the stress response, but also clear your mind of any obsessive or negative thought your guilt is producing.

- Close your eyes if possible. (I always carry an eye mask as darkness helps me.) Consciously release any tension in your body. Check that your face, jaw, hands, arms, legs and feet are loose. If you have time, you can also squeeze and release each set of muscles. Allow yourself to sink into, and feel supported by, whatever surface you are sitting or lying on.
- While mentally following the passage of your breath as it goes in and out, take three or four slow, deep breaths. To make sure that your breathing engages your diaphragm, put one hand on your stomach so you can feel it rise as your breath enters. Hold your breath when your stomach feels full and count to four or six. Then purse your lips

and blow the breath out as slowly as you can. Sometimes it helps to imagine your breath as one colour as it is drawn in and another as it is expelled.
- Now let yourself breathe naturally and easily, while slowly counting backwards from 50. Or, if you are not a numbers person, repeat the alphabet like this: ab ... bc ... cd ... de ... ef ... etc. Each time a thought enters your mind return to counting from 50 or repeating the alphabet exercise from the start.
- Finish by allowing your mind to just gently float for a few minutes. Your body should also feel light and loose.
- Repeat, if you have time.

SCENIC SYMBOL MEDITATION

This exercises tricks your brain into 'thinking' you are in your favourite tranquil place where you instantly feel relaxed. It works because our brains cannot distinguish between a scene we are really seeing and one that we are using our imagination to view.

- Relax your body by doing a few quick stretches of your muscles.
- Close your eyes and take three deep, slow breaths.
- Focus your mind's eye on your tranquil scene.
- Examine this scene in detail. Imagine that you are taking a video. Zoom in and out gently to take in all its beautiful details.
- Then use your mind's eye to watch this video. As you do, recall the scents and sounds, however faint they may be.
- Notice the positive sensations that have been created within your body. Take a few moments to enjoy them.
- Every time a thought comes into your head, refocus your mind's eye on some detail of your scene and examine it again carefully.

If you practise this technique regularly, you will teach your brain to associate the image of your scene with turning off the stress response. Then, when you notice a guilty thought, all you will need to do is bring this image to mind and your pulse rate will start to slow down.

Quick fixes for anxiety and fear

Fear is the enemy of logic.

FRANK SINATRA, AMERICAN SINGER AND ACTOR

Obviously all the above exercises will help you with anxiety and fear, too. Use them in conjunction with these suggestions below.

REASSURING SELF-TALK

- Write down a number of reassuring phrases on a small card that you can carry in your wallet or purse. Here are some examples of ones that have been used in different situations when fear or anxiety has joined up with guilt:

  I can handle this guilt.
  I am in control of my fear.
  I will focus on doing my very best.
  I can and will repair this situation. There is nothing to fear.
  I am not perfect. I am human.
  I cope better when I'm calm.
  I can postpone and prepare; I will have a good strategy/script.
  It will be a challenge, but I will have a reward even if it fails.
  I can make a contingency plan to deal with that.
  Only a small part of this mistake is my fault. Stay calm to think it through.

- Do one of the previous exercises to calm down your stress response.
- Take out your card and select a couple of reassuring phrases. Say these to yourself at least three times. Repeat whenever an anxious or fearful thought comes into your mind. If none of the phrases on your card seem suitable, write at least one or two that work for you.

IMAGINE PHONING A FRIEND

In certain game shows, when people are stuck for an answer (often because they are anxious) they are allowed to phone a friend for help. You may not be able to do this in reality, but you could do it in your imagination. The effect on your fear would be more or less the same.

- Bring to mind your favourite comedian. Imagine them whispering in your ear about this situation until you feel yourself smile or even laugh.
- Or recall someone you know or know about who is not, or was not, perfect and was willing to admit their guilt and move on positively. Imagine what they would say to you in this situation, which is making you anxious as well as guilty. (One person I used for many years was Nelson Mandela; another was a good friend. Many of my clients have chosen one of their grandparents.)
- Practise this exercise using different people. When you have chosen one or two, get a small photo of them to take around and look into their eyes when you begin to feel fearful. If you can't get hold of a photo, select a very small object that could represent them and that you could carry around with you or have on your desk.

SIMULATE HANDLING YOUR FEAR SUCCESSFULLY

Before you are about to do something in relation to the guilt that is inducing fear or anxiety, do this exercise. It works because we are less frightened about doing things that we have done several times before. Our brain cannot distinguish between what we have imagined and what has actually taken place. So we use our mind's eye to take us through a successful simulation. Examples of when this technique might be very useful would be:

- You are about to meet an ex whom you hurt by ending the relationship.
- You are going to a work conference where you will meet ex-colleagues who were made redundant from your company last year.

- You are a doctor and need to tell a patient that you made a mistake with their diagnosis last year. Recent tests show that the symptoms they had reported were unfortunately indicating a more serious condition.
- You are a manager who has been given the job of telling employees that 50 per cent of them will lose their jobs in three months' time.
- You have resolved to tell your partner that you lied last week about where you were one evening.

• • •

- Go somewhere very comfortable and quiet where you can lie down or sit. Ideally, you might choose to do this in a warm (not hot) bath.
- Do an exercise that will ensure you are in as relaxed a state as possible. At the very least, do some deep, slow breathing.
- Close your eyes and visualise yourself entering the scenario that you fear. Visualise yourself looking cool, calm and confident. Watch yourself doing what it is you want to do, or must do, superbly well.
- Watch yourself leaving, looking pleased and relieved and then phoning a friend to share with them how it went. Imagine them asking you questions about how you coped with your fears: *What did you say when ...?; How did you keep you cool when he said that?* Give them your answers.
- Repeat this visualisation three times over the few days just before your event.

Dealing with irritation and anger

'Come back!' the Caterpillar called after her. 'I've something important to say.'

This sounded promising, certainly. Alice turned and came back again.

'Keep your temper,' said the Caterpillar.

FROM *ALICE'S ADVENTURES IN WONDERLAND* BY LEWIS CARROLL

Anger is a very strong and dangerous emotion, but it can be very energising and useful when it is under your control. When it is triggered, our brain prepares us physiologically for a physical 'fight'. Our 'opponents' will automatically sense that we are doing this, and their auto-defence responses will switch on. So it is vital that we switch off this response during the very early stages of irritation. The Don't Get Too Boiling quick fix below has been tested out over many years and has proved extremely effective.

For those of you who feel and act out anger frequently, it is important that you seek more help with this problem. The combination of guilt and anger renders us liable to be very volatile. My book *Managing Anger*, which is a self-help programme, is a good place to start, but there are now also many anger-management courses available as well. Your doctor or local social services should be able to advise you on a reputable one in your area.

THE DON'T GET TOO BOILING STRATEGY: A QUICK FIX FOR RISING IRRITATION AND ANGER

This strategy can be used in a wide variety of situations, both at home and at work. It is also very useful when you are making difficult telephone calls and start to feel irritated (for example, when someone is goading you humorously about a mistake you made, but you sense that there is a critical undertone, you may find it hard to quell your irritation).

The four stages are each designed to send signals to the brain to say that you are no longer in danger and you do not need to fight. How you apply it will depend on a variety of factors, such as the degree of irritation or anger you are feeling, the place you are in, and whether or not you are able to physically leave the situation that has triggered your anger response. It can be used in a few moments if all you are feeling is irritation. If you are truly angry, the stages can, and should, be spaced out over hours or days.

Use this mnemonic to help you remember the stages and their order:

Don't	Get	Too	Boiling
I	R	E	R
S	O	N	E
T	U	S	A
A	N	I	T
N	D	O	H
C		N	E
E			

- **D**istance

The aim of this response is to create some distance between you and the person or situation that has aroused your irritation. In taking this step, you are in effect doing the same as animals do when they don't want to fight. (Dogs walk backwards when another dog is being aggressive and they don't want to fight.) This step will automatically send a 'back-off' message to your brain and to anyone involved.

Action: Let go of any physical contact you may have; take a step back; lean back in a chair; leave the room. If you are very angry and have time, do what Grandma suggests: *Sleep on it.*

- **G**round

Your aim in this step is to bring your body and mind back down to earth. Anger has a habit of making us move about threateningly. It can also make us think fantastically. This step grounds us both physically and mentally by taking our brain into its thinking mode (instead of being in its auto-emotional mode, which guilt ignites).

Action: Put both feet firmly on the ground; take hold of some firm inanimate object such as a desk, table bedpost or window ledge; count all the blue (or any colour) objects in the room or the number of circles you can see. Alternatively, distract yourself by thinking through a recipe for tonight's meal or doing a mundane, easy chore that requires concentration.

- **T**ension

The aim of this step is to release the physical tension that your anger response has created.

Action: If you can find a private spot such as a loo, screw up your face and release it slowly, and do some stretches and shake your wrists. If you are at home you could thump or kick a cushion, and even scream and let out a long, satisfying growl! If you have time, go to the gym or have a brisk walk or run.

Should you be in an important meeting, you can discreetly curl and uncurl toes or clench and unclench fists under the table.

- **B**reathe

Anger makes us hyperventilate so it is crucial to consciously do some controlled breathing to correct this. Hyperventilation is not only bad for us physically, it can also cause a panic attack and render us immobile and unable to function.

Action: Pause for a moment, breathe deeply into your stomach area and let the air out slowly. If you can take time out, do the exercise on pages 99–101. Continue to take a few deep, slow breaths over the next 3–5 minutes.

If you think you could do with a little more help with emotional management, some of my other books, such as *Emotional Confidence*, *Managing Anger* and *The Emotional Healing Strategy*, should help. Alternatively there are now many courses available on this subject. These will give you an opportunity to test out skills and techniques. This is the best way of finding the ones that work for you.

In the last decade or so, science has discovered a tremendous amount about the role emotions play in our lives. Researchers have found that, even more than IQ, your emotional awareness and abilities to handle feelings will determine your success and happiness in all walks of life.

JOHN GOTTMAN, AMERICAN PROFESSOR EMERITUS IN PSYCHOLOGY

Skill 5: Face-to-face friendship

The apparently cynical Ogden Nash quote opposite is actually a very wise comment. Guilt can be a very good test of friendship. It is often a maker or breaker. If you have done something that a friend disapproves of, they may not be able to forgive you, whatever you do or say. And if you are someone who is continually feeling guilty or is stuck fast in a guilt trip, you may find that some of your friends feel like seeing much less of you.

On the other hand, when guilt is crushing our self-esteem and joie de vivre, a certain friend may be the only rock we have to cling on to. Or we might lean on others who don't necessarily understand or accept our feelings, but who nevertheless stay loyally with us through whatever we do.

This morning I was listening to a piece on the radio about happiness. With good reason, this has become a hot topic in the Western world. More and more studies are now being published and each purports to shed new light on the subject. Most of the ones I have seen seem to agree on the importance of having a strong social network. And yet, it seems, fewer and fewer people feel that they have this. They may have hundreds or even thousands of social media contacts and many acquaintances, but few – if any – friends they would entrust with a guilty secret. I do not mean guilt over eating too much chocolate cake or allowing harmless flirtations. You can talk to a fellow bus passenger about these issues. But fewer and fewer people have enough friends or family with whom they can get support to help them through a more difficult personal problem.

My experience as a therapist certainly bears this out. I see many clients who just want to talk to me as they would talk to a friend face-to-face about their guilt issues. They just need a listening ear and a little reassurance that they are an okay person leading an okay life. They do not need therapy. So I am often giving them some guidance on making and developing closer relationships. The obvious advantages for my client are that friends are more available and their time doesn't cost money. The less obvious advantages are that, as friendship is a mutually caring relationship, we can reciprocate. Doing this helps to boost our confidence, is emotionally healing for the giver and, of course, deepens relationships that can last a lifetime.

> **There are people who are very resourceful at being remorseful, and who apparently feel that the best way to make friends is to do something terrible and then make amends.**
>
> OGDEN NASH, AMERICAN POET

Unfortunately, there are no quick and easy ways to make these kinds of face-to-face friendships. They take time to build and test out. But it does help if we know the personal qualities that we are seeking. Perhaps one day someone will produce a psychological test for potential friends, such as those used in job interviews. But who would want to use it? Can you imagine sitting down with a new acquaintance in a pub and saying, '*I think we could become really close friends, but would you mind completing this questionnaire first, please?*' This exercise is designed to help you do this if you are short on these kinds of friends.

EXERCISE: QUALITIES TO LOOK FOR IN FRIENDS TO HELP ME WITH GUILT

Below is a list that I have made. Look at it and personalise it to suit your needs. Add or subtract the qualities that you would like in friends to help you with a guilt issue. For example, if your guilt issues tend to be around work, you may want someone who understands your work culture. If they tend to be around parenting, you may need them to be a parent.

My examples list is a little over-long. For practical purposes, cut yours down to about six. Once your list is as you wish it to be, beside each entry write the names of your friends whom you know have at least some of the qualities you need. Ideally you need at least **two** people for each quality, as one might not be available.

- An ability to keep confidences.
- Similar core values.
- Open-mindedness.
- Positive outlook.
- Resilience – bounces back and doesn't normally become overpowered by problems.
- Confident enough to share their own failings.
- Respect for people who have different beliefs.
- Assertive enough to say 'No' to you when they want or need to do so.
- Good enough self-esteem to accept that you need other friends as well.
- A sense of humour to give perspective when things get a bit too 'heavy'.

An ability to love an imperfect person who is trying to improve!

Choose one or two friendships that you would like to deepen. Note down ways in which you could check out if they have any other of your key qualities, e.g. by starting specific conversations with them, noticing how they react to film subjects or what storylines they look for in their TV viewing, etc.

Of course, once we have selected our friends we have to be able to keep the relationship in good shape. That means doing the obvious, like spending quality time together. But it also means courageously dealing with problems that arise between you, and not just sweeping them under the carpet. This is so much easier said than done, however confident you are. So I have written a few guidelines, which I hope will help you to deal with common difficulties in relation to guilt within friendships. These have been based mainly on the knowledge I have gained over many years of working with clients in groups as well as in one-to-ones. And, of course, I have also drawn a good deal of wisdom from my own personal experience.

How to avoid crossed wires that result in guilt in face-to-face friendships

Crossed wires are sometimes caused by faulty communication skills, but in the area of friendship these are almost always due to misunderstood expectations. And these are responsible for most of the guilt that ensues.

In our working lives, we have contracts and job definitions. The expectations of the roles we play are usually clearly defined. Before people get married nowadays, expectations are also more often than not discussed. Rarely is this the case within the realm of friendships. Not surprisingly, this leads to many misunderstandings and a good deal of bad feeling between friends. It is unrealistic to think that expectations will ever be formally clarified between friends, but we can minimise the feelings of guilt and disappointment on both sides. Here are some suggestions:

Be clear about your own friendship needs and review them from time to time. They do change, especially as we and our friends age or go through transitional or stressful periods in our lives. Our needs can vary enormously. Here are just some of the common ones:

- Emotional support – people who truly care about me and respect my feelings.
- Practical mutual help.
- Having fun together.
- Being able to be fully ourselves.
- Having a confidante I can trust.
- Loyalty – having someone by my side.
- Having someone to challenge and stretch me.
- Having someone who shares my values.
- Being with people who are different from me.
- Having someone with whom to share adventures.
- Having people around who have been with me throughout most of my life.
- Playing and/or doing sport together.

Most of us cannot ever get our friendship needs fully met by one or two people. Neither can we get them met by one group of friends who always socialise together because they like doing the same activities. We have to have a selection and be clear in our own minds about what needs we think each of them can realistically meet.

Be honest and realistic about what you can and want to give in relation to each of your friends. Sensitively decline requests for help or activities if they are not in this list. If your friend persists in asking for what you do not want to do, use scripting (see page 90) to prepare something assertive to say to her or him.

Stop thinking in hierarchical terms about your friends – from best friend through to marginal friend. This will prevent you from having too high expectations of best friends and too low for the others. Think instead in terms of matching strengths to both of your needs at any one time.

Don't be afraid to change an activity that you habitually do with a friend. For example, Carole had a single friend from her college days who used to be a great person to go on shopping excursions with. Now she is a parent and also has a higher income, she feels guilty about dragging her into toy and baby departments and shops that sell clothes she cannot afford. She's arranged with her to have monthly cinema evenings, which gives them both much more enjoyment and satisfaction.

Avoid white lies as much as you can – they cause guilt. Eventually you will be found out and your guilt will be mountainous! Better to be assertive and use the Broken Record technique (see page 119) for pushy friends.

Double-check arrangements to avoid misunderstandings. I went through a phase a year ago when I failed to turn up on three occasions to meet the same friend! I was mortified by guilt. Now I always send a written message saying, *'Looking forward to seeing you next xx at xx in xx.'* I do this after making a date on the phone and a few days before we are due to meet. I have also set a reminder on my phone and computer. So far so good since I started this habit!

Keep clear boundaries if your friend is a colleague or client. This is easier said than done, but it is essential to try our very best to make sure this happens. Friendships at work get into hot, murky water when, for example, one person gets a promotion, a client has to be dropped for business reasons or one person gets made redundant. Guilt inevitably comes into play. It may not be rational, but it is still hard to feel and deal with. You will need even firmer boundaries for a while. It may also be best to decrease or cease friendship contact for an initial period until you have both had time to settle into your new working relationship. Unless you do this, feelings could interfere with your work and make matters worse. If you are the one feeling the guilt, analyse it using the DREAM Repair Kit (see Chapter 5) and talk through your feelings with a clear-headed friend. When you do see your colleague again as a friend, discuss your relationship – don't avoid doing so, even though that is tempting. You need to review your expectations and boundary lines. Don't discuss the guilt. The person feeling that should deal with it outside the relationship. It is their issue. Amends are probably not appropriate, but celebrating the renewal of the friendship certainly is!

If you have done something that you know is wrong, own up quickly – the results of not doing so are staple food for films, plays and TV dramas, and yet who learns? I am not talking about breaking the odd glass when we are helping to clear the table or even spilling red wine on their Chinese carpet. These misdemeanours do produce guilt but are relatively easy to deal with. Most of us would own up and make amends as best we could. I was referring to doing something that you know could, or definitely will, upset or hurt a friend, and then feeling so guilty that you repeatedly put off confessing. This could vary in its seriousness and may or may not be forgivable. Everyday examples would be breaking a confidence, smacking one of their children or having a one-night stand with their partner. Wrongful as these are, it is often the delay and '*carrying on as though nothing happened*' that hurts a friend the most. This can bring the offender an unsustainable burden of guilt. Make a confident apology as soon as you can. Use my strategy on page 90 to get the conversation going.

Give these friendships the real-life time that they need. Most of us nowadays communicate a good deal with our friends electronically. This is especially so if, like me, you have travelling lifestyles. I find that e-communication is responsible for many crossed wires. People are constantly asking me to read between the lines of texts and emails that friends have sent them. I confess to trying to do that as well in my personal e-communications.

But perhaps more importantly, the kind of friendships we need to help each other with guilt and deal with difficult issues do, I believe, require us to meet as often as we can in person. We need to be able to sense each other's feelings, touch each other, link arms, have hugs and sometimes just sit together in silence. New means of e-communication through social networking and video messaging are a great invention, and do meet some important needs, but I have never met anyone yet who believes that they are as satisfying or as bonding as real-life meetings.

If your wires become persistently tangled, cut them dead. I am afraid there is no pain-free way to do this. Do it quickly and firmly. Start with an appreciation; say the relationship just isn't working for you any longer so you are going to pull out. Don't get into giving explanations – they will be misunderstood and there will be more hurt. Don't get into blaming them or yourself. Stay focused on the fact that the relationship is not working for you (even if they plead that it still is for them!).

Sounds hard? It is. But in my experience it is still the best way forward for you both. Treat yourself afterwards and talk through the experience with someone who will understand and does not think you should feel guilty!

If you are now thinking that you could never manage to do this face-to-face, it is okay to do it in writing. That is better than not doing it. Choose an appropriate greetings card and send it by post. This is not a message that should ever be sent by text. If you are on the other side of the globe, use email or traditional post.

Using the Three Ps strategy for saying 'No' to a friend who drains your energy

Many of the techniques and strategies that I have included in this book will help you to develop and manage the face-to-face friendships you need. But there is a problem between friends that I am probably asked for advice on more than most. Even very confident people find it very hard to say 'No' to friends.

People who feel too much guilt are usually very kind, sensitive people. They care about the feelings and welfare of others. They are the type of people others want as friends, so they always have too many. And this means that they feel permanently guilty because they can't give them each enough time. As they are ever ready with a listening ear, they are an obvious choice when someone needs help. They rarely say 'No'. When they do *'have to'*, they feel unreasonably guilty. They will bend over backwards to make amends by giving them more time than usual.

So what's wrong with that, you may ask? Nothing, of course – as long it doesn't become the complete story of your life. Unfortunately, it often does. You can become trapped by your 'niceness' and your fear of guilt. You can spend so much time with friends who drain you that you have no time left for friends who energise you. I used to be no exception, and still sometimes struggle with this issue. This next example illustrates my favourite method of dealing with this self-sabotaging habit.

MY 'SAYING NO' STORY:

I am off to my house in Spain for a much-needed rest break. A friend, Jill, rings me. She is not someone I feel particularly close to. She can be fun, but she is very lively and I really didn't want to spend a day of my precious rest time with her. I have other, closer friends I wanted to see and needed to catch up with. As soon as she mentioned she was coming to Seville for the first time and would love to meet up, I knew I needed to use my **Three Ps strategy**. (I introduced this earlier on page 89.)

1. Postponement

Action: Stop yourself from answering the request. Steal some time to think and prepare your response.

Jill: Hi, Gael. I've heard that you're going to your house near Seville for a few weeks in December. I have booked a holiday in Seville at the same time. I am so excited. I have never been before. I thought we could meet up and you can show me the hidden sights, and I'll treat you to lunch.

Gael: Jill, can I ring you back tomorrow morning? I can't talk right now.

Jill: Okay. I'll be in from 9 to 10am.

Gael: Great. Speak tomorrow.

2. Preparation

Action: Think about the other person's relevant personality traits and feelings. Think about your own needs and feelings.

My mental notes: Jill is very persuasive. She's going to be so disappointed. I will feel sorry for her. I must stay focused on my need to have a restful break. Jill is fun but very lively. I must resist rescuing her by asking someone else to meet up with her instead: the reality is that she is an experienced traveller. She didn't consult me before booking this trip. I have a right to say 'No'. My other friends there are my priority.

I could easily give in, so I decide that I will need to use the Broken Record technique to help me persist with my decision (see page 119). I will need to empathise with her disappointment.

I must also do some quick stretches and deep breathing and make sure I have breakfast before calling. I don't want to get irritated.

3. Practice

Action: Choose your 'Broken Record' phrase (if that is the strategy you choose). Write out what you will say at first and then plan your replies to anything your friend might say in response. Do some relaxation stretches and deep breathing before you speak. You must be relaxed to sound confident and convincing. Rehearse what you have planned to say, using a brisk, confident tone.

Here's how my Broken Record phrase (i.e. '... ***going to say "no"*** *...'*) was used:

Gael: Hi, Jill. How great that you have booked a trip to Seville. I know you will love it.

Jill: Yes, I am so pleased you are doing a Spain trip then. I would love to see the 'real' city and not just the obvious tourist sights. I am likely to end up lost if I just try to wander off-piste by myself.

Gael: Jill, I am going to Spain for a rest so I am **going to say 'no'** this time.

Jill: Oh no! I was banking on seeing you there. We haven't had a catch-up for ages. John knows Seville but he can't come. Surely you can come just for a night? I will treat you to the hotel and dinner. It is in a very peaceful location.

Gael: That's very kind of you but I am still **going to say 'no'**.

Jill: We can take it very easy, and I know you love Seville.

Gael: It is a lovely idea and a generous offer. I guess you are disappointed, but I am still **going to say 'no'**.

Jill: When are you going back? I could perhaps pop over and see you one day.

Gael: Jill, I am **going to say 'no'** to that as well. I want to have a good rest.

Jill: Well, yes, I <u>am</u> disappointed, but it's okay! Enjoy your rest. I know you deserve it. I guess I'll survive being solo in Seville. Perhaps we can meet up some time in London next year!

Gael: Okay. I'll let you know when I have some free time. Enjoy Seville, Jill.

BROKEN RECORD

Broken Record is the name of an assertiveness technique, which consists of repeating a brief key statement over and over again until the person accepts your point or gives you what you want, or you reach a compromise you can accept.

- You choose a key brief phrase that sums up the main message you want to get across.
- Each time the other person says something to persuade you to change your mind, repeat your phrase.
- You can use it on its own or you can 'soften' your message a little by wrapping a brief sentence around it. You can also vary one or two words so you don't sound too much like a parrot.
- When using it with a friend or someone in a low power position, it is sensible and kind to also include an empathy sentence, which shows that you have thought about their feelings and/or situation.
- Do not get side-tracked by comments designed to pull at your heartstrings, seduce you or threaten you.
- Do not answer unnecessary or revealing questions.
- Ensure that your body language, including your tone of voice, conveys confidence.

EXERCISE: THE THREE PS AND BROKEN RECORD

- Choose an example that could be a real-life request challenge to you. Or think of a hypothetical one. Work through the first two steps of the Three Ps, including writing out a Broken Record script.
- Try out the script for yourself with a friend, or use two chairs – one for your friend and one for you. Move between the two as you act out your script. The harder you make these practice sessions, the easier your real-life ones will become.
- Soon after you have used your Broken Record in real life, give yourself a reward! You have done something that is very difficult to do.

If it's very painful for you to criticise your friends – you're safe in doing it. But if you take the slightest pleasure in it, that's the time to hold your tongue.

ALICE MILLER, PSYCHOTHERAPIST AND AUTHOR

Updating my face-to-face friendship network

Finally, as I said earlier, our friendship circles are ever evolving and guilt is a great test of friendship. If you begin to feel that you do not seem to have enough people to turn to whom you truly trust and to whom you could turn to with your dark thoughts, it is time to review your friendships.

Don't wait until you really need the type of friends who could help you; that would not be a good time to go hunting for one. Some of these kinds of friendships take time to build. You may not have to search for completely new people – you may only need to spend more quality time with some you already know. Remember, to help support you when you feel guilty you may need help from a diverse set of friends.

This next exercise will clarify the specific qualities and abilities you will be looking for.

EXERCISE: REVIEW OF MY FACE-TO-FACE FRIENDSHIPS

Make a list of your main face-to-face friends – noting down the following beside each:

a) What are your main expectations from the friendship, and are they met?
b) Do you think these expectations are shared or do you think this friend may have different ones? Is this a subject you could discuss together?
c) What are your main contributions to the friendship? Does your friend appreciate these?
d) Which kinds of issues would you not feel okay discussing with them?
e) Are there any outstanding guilt issues between you? If so, how could these be resolved?
f) Write yourself an action plan (see Chapter 9 for templates). Be specific about what you need to do and when and how you will do it. If you need extra time to make new face-to-face friendships or to deepen existing ones, how would you find it (e.g. perhaps by cutting back on the time you spend on social networking websites/giving up a class you go to/cutting down on the time you spend on a hobby or sport)?

You can't stay in your corner of the Forest waiting for others to come to you. You have to go to them sometimes.

FROM *WINNIE-THE-POOH* BY A. A. MILNE

CHAPTER 5

The DREAM Repair Kit

The DREAM Repair Kit is a strategy and a set of tools that you can use to analyse your guilt and plan constructive action. The actual process of doing this will help you to stay in control of your guilt feelings. This is because, in order to work through this strategy, you will need to engage the logical-thinking centre in your brain – the neocortex region. The feeling part of your brain – the amygdala – has done its job. It alerted you to the fact that you have been operating on shaky moral ground. Like all emotional responses, its purpose was to get you into action.

If at this stage you do not consciously and quickly engage your thinking brain, your emotional brain will kick you into its own kind of action. It will trigger the primitive fight/flight/freeze response, which we looked at in Chapter 4. If this should happen, you would either become angrily defensive, run away or do nothing. As you know, people who get caught in guilt traps usually do nothing (i.e. they 'freeze'). This is why they become stuck with their guilty feelings

The fight response commonly makes us lay the blame on others:

- *He was the leader; I was just following his orders.*
- *You shouldn't have looked at me like that. You started it.*

- *If you had put your bike away as you should, I wouldn't have smashed it up.*
- *You're never here now; is it any wonder I was so easily seduced?*
- *If I'm selfish, whose fault is it? You brought me up!*

The flight response (i.e. denial or disassociation in today's humans) may temporarily sort the problem. But as we saw when looking at disguised guilt in Chapter 2, that can play havoc with our physical and psychological health. There is also the danger that it could burst through in sarcasm and anger. It would then do similar damage to that of the fight response.

The result of the freeze response (often caused by suppressed guilt, i.e. awareness but doing nothing, or disguised guilt, i.e. denial) readers of this book will likely know about all too well! Experience has taught us that the more we hide guilt, the harder it becomes to 'out' it. Mercy will be in short supply because of our deception. Our 'punishment', therefore, will be far greater than our 'sin' would have originally merited. Our relationship with the person we hurt may also become irreparable. A break in trust is extremely hard and often impossible to mend. Using the DREAM Repair kit is, as I hope you will agree, a more positive option.

Playing for time

As with most other strategies for solving problems where emotions are running high, we need first to play for time in order to be able to use the kit. You can do this by following these three steps:

1. **Apologise**: *I'm really very sorry to have hurt you/broken the plate/let you down/not kept our promise/broken the contract/deceived you for so long/not visited for so long/the project wasn't the success we anticipated.*
2. **Postpone**: *I need to finish off what I am doing/gather some information/have some time with you alone/discuss the issue with my boss and colleagues before we talk about this.*

3. **Rearrange**: *Can we arrange a time to talk later?/I am available tomorrow morning or Saturday/we can discuss it fully at our meeting.*

Depending on the complexity or seriousness of the issue, using the DREAM Repair Kit can take several minutes, several hours or days. In the hands of guilty organisations, similar strategies may take months or even years (for fraudulent practice, oil spills or war enquiries, for example)!

Obviously, if you think it is going to take longer than the hurt people wish, you will once again need to summon up your assertiveness skills. You could use **scripting** (page 90) to help you start a negotiation. Don't forget to empathise with their frustration and point out the positive side of doing a thorough investigation. If they keep persisting in their attempts to speak immediately, just use the **Broken Record strategy** (page 119) until they stop. (They will!)

Overview of the DREAM Repair Kit

There are five templates to work through in the kit. Before the questions there is a summary of the overall task to achieve when completing each of them. Then there are examples of how the five templates have been used to analyse and plan action for a couple of guilt issues. Once you have become practised at using the five DREAM steps you should not need the templates, unless the issue is quite complicated. The idea is that you will use the kit to establish a new good habit to manage your guilt. This one will replace the bad one that has been trapping the guilt within you.

After my explanation of the process, I will give you some examples of how you can use the kit with a number of different guilt issues.

The word DREAM is a mnemonic to help you remember these five stages.

1. **D**amage assessment
2. **R**esponsibility pie chart

3. **E**thics review
4. **A**mends to arrange
5. **M**anagement tools for feelings

The kit can be used for any type of guilt. It can be about something that:

a) you know you have done or omitted to do that was wrong;
b) was a wrongdoing or omission that you know you are partly responsible for;
c) you are worried you may deserve to feel guilty about for an action or non-action in the past;
d) you would deserve if you did something or omitted to do something in the future;
e) someone else whom you are helping (such as your child or a friend) has done or not done.

To keep the wording of the strategy simple and concise, I have written the following explanations and templates as if we are dealing with type a. If you wanted to use a template for any of the other options you would only need to alter a little of the wording. For example, for use with type c you could change '**Task:** To assess the hurt that **has been** done ...' to: '**Task:** To assess the hurt that **might have been** done ...'

The tasks of the five steps remain essentially the same for all types of guilt, even though the action you take to deal with them may be different.

TEMPLATES

In completing your answers in these templates, mark any fact or feeling that hasn't been, or cannot be, proven with a question mark. Alternatively, you could just highlight the facts.

Remember, these templates are for your personal use only. You are not being cross-examined in a court of law; you are just making 'guesstimates' to help you with your task of managing your guilt.

The DREAM Repair Kit templates

1. DAMAGE ASSESSMENT

Task: To assess the hurt that has been done as a result of the wrongdoing. This could be a fact, or something you have surmised or heard or read about.

Note down as specifically as possible the damage that has been, or will be, done. This could be to you as well as to other people or to property or other things.

a) Physical (e.g. a wound or damage to a car, beloved object, etc.).

....

....

....

....

b) Psychological (e.g. self-esteem, sense of security, loneliness, reputation).

....

....

....

....

c) Financial (e.g. loss of money or valuable object).

....

....

....

....

d) Any other.

....

....

....

....

....

....

2. Responsibility Pie Chart

Task: To assess as accurately as you can your share of the responsibility for the wrongdoing. To help you do this you will first need to look at the responsibility that other people and other factors may share.

a) List the people (or groups of people, such as a department or a family) who were involved. They could be implicated directly (e.g. a colleague or brother) or indirectly (e.g. a shareholder or your supervisor).

....

....

....

....

....

....

....

....

b) List other factors that may have played a part as well (e.g. weather, austerity, traffic chaos).

....

....

....

....

....

....

c) Decide the percentage of the total responsibility attributable to each of the people or factors involved.

....

....

....

....

....

....

....

d) If possible, talk this over with a friend who is preferably a logical thinker (rather than one who would feel sorry for you!). Show them your list and amend it if they have convinced you to think differently. If you prefer to do this on your own, write a short description of what happened and why you have apportioned out the responsibility as you have. Use the GEE or Three Cs strategies (on pages 85 and 87) to check that the thinking you have used to write the description is rational and is not being skewed by your guilt.

....

....

....

....

....

....

....

....

....

....

....

....

....

e) Now, finally, you are ready to draw your pie chart. You will need to roughly estimate the percentage of responsibility that each of the people and factors involved carries. Don't forget to include yourself, of course! Imagine that you have to 'cut' a pie into pieces. Each piece will reflect the amount of responsibility each person or factor shares for this wrongdoing. Then draw a picture that shows the size of each piece. Nowadays, you can get a computer to draw your pie chart, or you can simply draw a circle and use different coloured pens for each of the sections.

3. Ethics review

Task: To clarify your understanding of which of your own values you have disrespected when you engaged in this wrongdoing, and to check whether you have disrespected any other values, and then to give the wrongdoing an overall ethical rating.

Recall the list of the ten values that you considered to be most important for you and the three personal life rules that you made.

a) Note which of your own values and personal life rules were being disrespected or broken when you engaged in this wrongdoing.

....

....

....

b) Note whether you disrespected any organisational moral code, such as a law, a company's code of ethics, a religious code or an unwritten code (e.g. family values).

....

....

....

c) Note whether by doing what you did, or omitted to do, you were knowingly disrespecting someone else's values. (That someone should be someone for whom you do have respect, regard or love.)

....

....

....

d) Give this wrongdoing an overall ethical rating. For example, using a 1–10 scale, if you have been very unethical you might score 2/10, or if your moral compass has not been too off centre, your ethical score might be 8/10.

....

....

4) Amends to arrange

Task: To assess possible ways in which you could make amends to the victim(s) of your wrongdoing. This may first include finding out from the victim or someone who knows them well what kind of amends would be appropriate and acceptable.

a) Re-read your notes on step one, the **D**amage assessment. Note down your own ideas for making amends for each type of damage.

....

....

....

b) Look at your **R**esponsibility pie chart from step two. If others are partly responsible for the wrongdoing, note down if there is anything you could do to ensure that they deal with their share of the responsibility (e.g. talk to them, campaign for change, etc.).

....

....

....

c) Discuss your ideas with a friend who may be able to add some more ideas.

....

....

d) Prepare a concise proposal for your victim. It should include an **apology**, your **ideas for amends**, a request for their opinion and **alternative or additional ideas** and, finally, a **positive expression of hope** that these will go some way towards making recompense so you can move on.

Your initial proposal should not refer to other people's responsibility for the wrongdoing. If your amends have included trying to get others to deal with their responsibility, this would be best addressed later.

....

....

5) MANAGEMENT TOOLS FOR FEELINGS

Task: To clarify what residual feelings you may have about dealing with this issue, now or in the future. Identifying the strategies and tools you can use to help you manage them.

a) Note down any additional feelings, apart from guilt, that you have right now.

....

....

....

....

....

b) Note down any feelings you may have when presenting your amends proposal to the victim.

....

....

....

....

....

c) Note down any feelings that you could have when you move on from this incident.

....

....

....

....

....

d) Note down the tools or strategies you could use to help you manage these feelings. If they are in this book, note down the page number beside each.

....

....

....

....

....

The DREAM Repair Kit: Example 1

Angie is a divorced working mother with two teenage daughters – 15-year-old Trish and 17-year-old Arabella. A couple of months ago, the girls were spending a weekend with their father. While cleaning Arabella's room, Angie found a piece of paper with a funny name and a code for a password on it. Angie decided to note these things down. She told herself that if ever she became suspicious or worried about her daughter she might need them. After all, there were many stories circulating about young girls being groomed on the internet.

The following Saturday evening, both the girls were out and Angie saw that Arabella had left her laptop in the sitting room. All week Angie had been thinking about the password code she had found. She had come up with a few possibilities and couldn't resist trying them out on her laptop. One of her guesses worked. Among the websites in the computer's history she found a teen-chat site. The name and password worked, so she scrolled through her daughter's conversations. She found nothing that worried her and closed the laptop quite quickly.

But over the next week Angie's guilt about having done what she did began to haunt her. Trust between her and her daughters was a constant theme in their conversations, and now it was she who had broken it and not, as she had always feared, her daughters. After talking to a good friend, Angie decided she had to confess to Arabella. This is how she used the DREAM Repair Kit to prepare.

1. Damage assessment

Task: To assess the hurt that has been done as a result of the wrongdoing. This could be a fact, or something you have surmised or heard or read about.

Note down as specifically as possible the damage that has been, or will be, done. This could be to you as well as to other people or to property or other things.

a) Physical (e.g. a wound or damage to a car, beloved object, etc.).

...........N/A...

....

....

....

....

b) Psychological (e.g. self-esteem, sense of security, loneliness).

My self-esteem; trust between me and the girls, particularly Arabella. ....

....

....

....

c) Financial (e.g. loss of money or valuable object).

...........N/A...

....

....

....

....

d) Any other.

...........N/A...

....

....

....

....

2. Responsibility Pie Chart

Task: To assess as accurately as you can your share of the responsibility for the wrongdoing. To help you do this you will first need to look at the responsibility that other people and other factors may share.

a) List the people (or groups of people, such as a department or a family) who were involved. They could be implicated directly (e.g. a colleague or brother) or indirectly (e.g. a shareholder or your supervisor).

............N/A...
....
....
....
....

b) List some factors that may have played their part as well (e.g. weather, austerity, traffic chaos).

Divorce has made me overprotective? The internet stories – people who use it for grooming young girls. The media for hyping up the stories. I have been thinking a lot about them. ....
....
....
....
....
....

c) Decide the percentage of the total responsibility attributable to each of the people or factors involved.

Divorce: 5% ... Media stories: 10% ... Me: 85% ....
....
....
....
....
....

d) If possible, talk this over with a friend who is preferably a logical thinker (rather than one who would feel sorry for you!). Show them your list and amend it if they have convinced you to think differently. If you prefer to do this on your own, write a short description of what happened and why you have apportioned out the responsibility as you have. Use the GEE or Three Cs strategies (on pages 85 and 87) to check that the thinking you have used to write the description is rational and is not being skewed by your guilt.

Will talk over with my friend Moira – she has teens and is always so calm and confident. ....

....

....

....

....

....

....

e) Now, finally, you are ready to draw your pie chart. You will need to roughly estimate the percentage of responsibility that each of the people and factors involved carry. Don't forget to include yourself, of course! Imagine that you have to 'cut' a pie into pieces. Each piece will reflect the amount of responsibility each person or factor shares for this wrongdoing. Then draw a picture that shows the size of each piece. Nowadays, you can get a computer to draw your pie chart, or you can simply draw a circle and use different coloured pens for each of the sections.

3. Ethics review

Task: To clarify your understanding of which of your own values you have disrespected when you engaged in this wrongdoing, and to check whether you have disrespected any other values, and then to give the wrongdoing an overall ethical rating.

Recall the list of the ten values that you considered to be most important for you and the three personal life rules that you made.

a) Note which of your own values and personal life rules were being disrespected when you engaged in this wrongdoing.

Broke my rule number 1: To maintain a high quality of relationship with my daughters. Honesty and trust are top values for me.

....

....

....

....

....

....

....

....

b) Note whether you disrespected any organisational moral code, such as a law, a company's code of ethics, a religious code or an unwritten code (e.g. family values).

...........N/A...

....

....

....

....

....

....

....

....

....

c) Note whether by doing what you did, or omitted to do, you were knowingly disrespecting someone else's values. (That someone should be someone for whom you do have respect, regard or love.)

Arabella ... and indirectly Trish. ....
....
....
....
....
....
....
....

d) Give this wrongdoing an overall ethical rating. For example, using a 1–10 scale, if you have been very unethical you might score 2/10, or if your moral compass has not been too off centre, your ethical score might be 8/10.

5/10 ....
....
....
....
....
....
....
....
....

4) AMENDS TO ARRANGE

Task: To assess possible ways in which you could make amends to the victim(s) of your wrongdoing. This may first include finding out from the victim or someone who knows them well what kind of amends would be appropriate and acceptable.

a) Re-read your notes on step one, the **D**amage assessment, and note down your own ideas for making amends for each type of damage.

Take Arabella to London for a night to see a show and do some shopping. Have time to talk and emphasise my regret and promise never to do it again. Say how much I do trust her and feel so lucky to be able to do so. ....
....
....

b) Look at your **R**esponsibility pie chart from step two. If others are partly responsible for the wrongdoing, note down if there is anything you could do to ensure that they deal with their share of responsibility (e.g. talk to them, campaign for change, etc.).

Start a discussion on mumsnet.com about the issue of grooming stories and the fear they create. ....
....
....

c) Discuss your ideas with a friend who may be able to add some more ideas.

Have lunch with Moira and talk through. ....
....
....
....
....

d) Prepare a concise proposal for your victim. It should include an **apology**, your **ideas for amends**, a request for their opinion and **alternative or additional ideas** and, finally, a **positive expression of hope** that these will go some way towards making recompense so you can move on.

Your initial proposal should not refer to other people's responsibility for the wrongdoing. If your amends have included trying to get others to deal with their responsibility, this would be best addressed later.

I am so sorry, darling, but I want to tell you I have done something that I should never have done. I found your teen-chat password code and last Saturday used it to have a brief look through your conversations ... I know I have hurt you and you have a right to be angry. I do feel very guilty. Although now is not the time, I do so much want to find a way to make it up to you. I love you very, very much and am determined to rebuild your trust in me. ....
....
....
....
....
....
....
....
....
....
....
....
....
....
....
....
....
....
....
....

5) MANAGEMENT TOOLS FOR FEELINGS

Task: To clarify what residual feelings you may have about dealing with this issue, now or in the future. Identifying the strategies and tools you can use to help you to manage them.

a) Note down any additional feelings, apart from guilt, that you have right now.

Fear that I have done lasting damage to my relationship with both girls. ....

....

....

b) Note down any feelings you may have when presenting your amends proposal to the victim.

She will be so angry and won't listen ... I will use scripting as a guide to make sure I am concise. I may have to give it a couple of goes if she walks off. ....

....

....

c) Note down any feelings that you could have when you move on from this incident.

It could take a long time to get my relationship with Arabella back on track. I could start to get depressed about it. ....

....

....

d) Note down the tools or strategies you could use to help you manage these feelings. If they are in this book, note down the page number beside each.

Use the negative-thinking strategies (pages 80–88) and the calming ones (pages 99–108). ....

....

The DREAM Repair kit: Example 2

Brian was having a catch-up with a university friend, James, who told him that he was applying for a new job, which, he had heard through a contact, was coming up. Over the next few days Brian wondered if he should also apply for the job. He was currently working for a more prestigious company of accountants than the one James worked for. He knew, therefore, that his application might be treated more favourably. After tussling with the idea of telling James, he didn't. He thought that he would face the music if and when he was short-listed.

A week later he had an email from James saying that he had heard that someone from Brian's company had applied for the job and asking if he knew who it was.

After talking it through with his wife, Zelda, Brian decided he had to ring James. He promised himself he would do it at the weekend. In the meantime, he received a call from the company asking him to come for an interview. He was on the short-list. Brian felt even guiltier. He spent a couple of very uncomfortable days battling with his conscience and arguing with his wife about whether he should withdraw his application. He made up his mind to do this. Zelda was furious. They had decided to try for a baby and she said that they would need the extra money. She called Brian a coward and said he wasn't close to James anyway.

Brian later decided to leave his application in, as he knew Zelda was right about needing the extra money for the baby. But he did decide to tell James the truth in the hope that he could repair their relationship. This is the DREAM analysis he did in preparation.

1. Damage assessment

Task: To assess the hurt that has been done as a result of the wrongdoing. This could be a fact, or something you have surmised or heard or read about.

Note down as specifically as possible the damage that has been, or will be, done. This could be to you as well as to other people or to property or other things.

a) Physical (e.g. a wound or damage to a car, beloved object, etc.).

My tension headaches. ....
....
....
....

b) Psychological (e.g. self-esteem, sense of security, loneliness).

Self-esteem and confidence; insecurity about marriage after this clash of values with Zelda. ....
....
....

c) Financial (e.g. loss of money or valuable object).
............N/A..
....
....
....
....

d) Any other.

Breaking of a friendship; possible damage to reputation as local accountancy world is small. ....
....
....
....

2. Responsibility Pie Chart

Task: To assess as accurately as you can your share of the responsibility for the wrongdoing. To help you do this you will first need to look at the responsibility that other people and other factors may share.

a) List the people (or groups of people, such as a department or a family) who were involved. They could be implicated directly (e.g. a colleague or brother) or indirectly (e.g. a shareholder or your supervisor).

Zelda. ....

....

....

....

b) List other factors that may have played their part as well (e.g. weather, austerity, traffic chaos).

Financial pressure – austerity policies: salary increments being severely reduced; lack of promotional opportunities. ....

....

....

....

....

....

....

c) Decide the percentage of the total responsibility attributable to each of the people or factors involved.

Zelda: 15% ... Austerity: 10% ... Company cutbacks: 10% ... Me: 65% ...

....

....

....

....

d) If possible, talk this over with a friend who is preferably a logical thinker (rather than one who would feel sorry for you!). Show them your list and amend it if they have convinced you to think differently. If you prefer to do this on your own, write a short description of what happened and why you have apportioned out the responsibility as you have. Use the GEE or Three Cs strategies (on pages 85 and 87) to check that the thinking you have used to write the description is rational and is not being skewed by your guilt.

e) Now, finally, you are ready to draw your pie chart. You will need to roughly estimate the percentage of responsibility that each of the people and factors involved carry. Don't forget to include yourself, of course! Imagine that you have to 'cut' a pie into pieces. Each piece will reflect the amount of responsibility each person or factor shares for this wrongdoing. Then draw a picture that shows the size of each piece. Nowadays, you can get a computer to draw your pie chart, or you can simply draw a circle and use different coloured pens for each of the sections.

3. Ethics review

Task: To clarify your understanding of which of your own values you have disrespected when you engaged in this wrongdoing, and to check whether you have disrespected any other values, and then to give the wrongdoing an overall ethical rating.

Recall the list of the ten values that you considered to be most important for you and the three personal life rules that you made.

a) Note which of your own values and personal life rules were being disrespected when you engaged in this wrongdoing.

Loyalty and courage have always been top values for me. ....

....

b) Note whether you disrespected any organisational moral code, such as a law, a company's code of ethics, a religious code or an unwritten code (e.g. family values).

Unwritten but the expected friendship code about loyalty and trust?

....

c) Note whether by doing what you did, or omitted to do, you were knowingly disrespecting someone else's values. (That someone should be someone for whom you normally have respect, regard or love.)

James's trust – he would never have told me about the job if he thought I would do this. ....

....

d) Give this wrongdoing an overall ethical rating. For example, using a 1–10 scale, if you have been very unethical you might score 2/10, or if your moral compass has not been too off centre, your ethical score might be 8/10.

6/10 ....

4) Amends to arrange

Task: To assess possible ways in which you could make amends to the victim(s) of your wrongdoing. This may first include finding out from the victim or someone who knows them well what kind of amends would be appropriate and acceptable.

a) Re-read your notes on step one, the **D**amage assessment. Note down your own ideas for making amends for each type of damage.

Can try to get James into the company if I get the job; recommend him on LinkedIn. ....

....

....

....

....

....

b) Look at your **R**esponsibility pie chart from step two. If others are partly responsible, note down if there is anything you could do to ensure that they deal with their share of responsibility (e.g. talk to them, campaign for change, etc.).

Need to talk over what happened with Zelda. We were not on the same page with our values. ....

....

....

....

....

c) Discuss your ideas with a friend who may be able to add some more ideas.

............N/A..

....

....

....

....

d) Prepare a concise proposal for your victim. It should include an **apology**, your **ideas for amends**, a request for their opinion and **alternative or additional ideas** and, finally, a **positive expression of hope** that these will go some way towards making recompense so you can move on.

Your initial proposal should not refer to other people's responsibility for the wrongdoing. If your amends have included trying to get others to deal with their responsibility, this would be best addressed later.

....

....

....

....

....

....

....

....

....

....

Brian's script:

James, I have a big apology to make to you. I am the applicant from my company for the job. I know full well that I should have told you before I sent it, but I kept chickening out. That was cowardly.

I really am very sorry and am hoping I can make it up to you. If I do get the job, I will definitely see what I can do for you. In the meantime, I am doing a recommendation of you on LinkedIn. I know these are paltry amends for being so disloyal. Please let me know if there is ever anything I can do for you. I certainly owe you one and I won't forget that. This has taught me a big lesson. So I do hope eventually we can meet as friends again.

5) MANAGEMENT TOOLS FOR FEELINGS

Task: To clarify what residual feelings you may have about dealing with this issue, now or in the future. Identifying the strategies and tools you can use to help you manage them.

a) Note down any additional feelings, apart from guilt, that you have right now.

Shaky self-confidence, disappointment with myself. ....

....

....

....

....

....

....

....

b) Note down any feelings you may have when presenting your amends proposal to the victim.

Guilt and shame. ....

....

....

....

....

....

....

c) Note down any feelings that you could have when you move on from this incident.

Relief! But some anxiety about my marriage. ....

....

....

....

....

....

d) Note down the tools or strategies you could use to help you manage these feelings. If they are in this book, note down the page number beside each.

Am feeling negative; need to check it does not affect my decision making: GEE strategy or Three Cs? Pages 85 and 87. ....

....

....

....

....

....

....

....

....

....

....

....

....

....

....

....

....

....

Speedy use of the DREAM Repair Kit for guilt

As I said earlier, eventually you will not need to use the templates. If the wrongdoing has been relatively minor, you may be able to quickly run through the stages in your head. Doing so will calm your guilt feelings and help you take more effective action. But if you have time, I would also advise writing down your notes. The action of writing is more calming for the feelings, and seeing the words will fix them more firmly in your memory. Here's an example of how it can be used very quickly once you have had some practice.

EXAMPLE:

On her way home from a work meeting that ran late, Freda exceeded the speed limit. The cameras caught her and soon afterwards she received a fine. She hasn't told her husband Pete because he will 'go mad' at her. They have two children and their finances are stretched. She feels guilty for taking a risk that could have caused an accident and also for keeping it secret. Guilty thoughts have started to obsessively swirl around in her head. She feels shaky much of the time and keeps losing concentration at work. At lunchtime she makes these notes:

1. **D**amage: My confidence and stress; work performance; possible loss of trust if Pete finds out.
2. **R**esponsibility: 100% mine, even though meeting ran late.
3. **E**thics: V. bad – 2/10.
4. **A**mends: Will confess to Pete and say that I know I was very wrong to speed and keep it secret ... and will cancel the order for my new coat to pay the fine and promise not to do that again ... learned my lesson ... promise to drive safely whatever.
5. **M**anagement: Do relaxation before telling Pete and deep breathing in car when I feel tempted to speed. Ask kids to check me when they are in car.

EXERCISE: DREAM GUILT REPAIR

Choose something that either in the past or the present you feel guilty about. Use the templates to help you analyse your guilt and plan your action. As usual, if you can share what you have done with a friend and ask for comments, please do. Practise using the DREAM Repair Kit strategy as much as you can during the next few months so that it becomes embedded in your mind and you can use it quickly.

CHAPTER 6

Dealing with Guilt-tripping

What is guilt-tripping?

Perhaps as a reader of this book this is a question for which you don't need an answer. If you are someone for whom guilt is a big issue, you will already have been sniffed out as easy prey by those who excel at guilt-tripping. But for those of you who may be fortunate enough never to have experienced being tripped, I will clarify what I understand it to be. Guilt-tripping is an attempt to psychologically manipulate another person in order to make them feel guilty, so that they do what you want them to do or stop doing. In describing this behaviour in everyday language, people might say something like, *'She knows just how to push my buttons'* or *'He always makes me feel so guilty.'*

Those of us who are vulnerable to being influenced by this type of behaviour need to first and foremost remember the following:

- Guilt-tripping behaviour is aggressive.
- We have a right to protect ourselves from it.
- We do not have to accept the guilt.
- Assertive responses can usually stop the guilt-tripping behaviour.

One of the problems with this manipulative behaviour is that it can be hard to spot. This is because it is often mixed in with caring or flattering language and behaviour. We may be so used to it in certain relationships that we don't notice it until it has done its damage. This is particularly true if the relationship is one that dates back to our childhood, or is one in which we may be blinded by the respect or love that we have for the manipulating person.

So, the first step in protecting yourself is to sharpen your awareness of the signs that it is probably happening. Here are some common clues to look out for that act as warning signals. Of course, if you see one of them, that doesn't mean that the person is trying to guilt trip you. You need to watch out for a few different signals.

Guilt-tripping body language to watch out for

- Whining tone
- Sighing
- Lowered head
- Slightly shaking head
- Hand on head
- Tearful eyes
- Raised eyebrows
- Rolling eyes
- Sarcastic looks

Common types of guilt-tripping behaviour to notice

1. **Arriving with your favourite food or special presents before they ask a favour** – *'Here's some freshly baked ginger bites ... I know you're busy today, but could you just run me down to the station? Taxis are so expensive nowadays.'/'Hi, folks. Fresh doughnuts here for the taking! Who would mind staying over for an hour tonight? We have the regulators in next week and there's so much to catch up on. I don't know whether I'm coming or going. The finance department is breathing down my neck as well for the budget.'* (A boss to his team.)

2. **Flattering before delivering the stinging loaded comment** – *'You've done well, but money isn't everything, you know.'/'It's a beautiful flat ... so much bigger than we have ever had.'/'Well done for getting into uni. You are so lucky to be able to ...'*
3. **Being sick but carrying on or putting up with it 'bravely'** – *'Your poor father would go to work whether he was ill or not ...'/'I am not myself today, but don't worry, I'll pick them up as usual.'/'Okay, if you can't come in, you can't ... I had the bug last week and just powered through, but there we are.'*
4. **Comparing** – *'Some poor children are not lucky enough to have any food ... so finish your dinner!'/'Look at Charlie, he's not making a fuss.'/'Well done for getting into university. You're so lucky to be blessed with the brains ...'/'Did you know that Julia took her mum with her to Ibiza this year?'/'No one else leaves at 6pm on the dot.'*
5. **Suffering hardship gallantly** – *'We had to sacrifice our free time, but we didn't mind.'/'Glad to hear you're doing well. It's just under three years now since I got the push, but you have to make the best of the cards destiny deals you.'*
6. **Arousing sympathy to excuse hurtful or bad behaviour** – *'He was hard on you, but that was Dad's way of loving you.'/'I don't have a rich dad like you; I thought you wouldn't mind me borrowing a tenner.'*
7. **Questioning your financial decisions** – *'I grant you it's nice, but I heard that designer stuff is a rip-off and is all made in sweatshops.'/'Your organic food may taste better, but it costs a bomb. Most people can't afford it.'*
8. **Threatening future guilt** – *'When you are older you will appreciate that I can't do everything; you'd be sorry if my heart gave out.'/'Well, it's your choice who you hire, but don't say I didn't warn you.'/'I think that's an overly risky strategy. If we lose this contract, it will be on your shoulders.'*
9. **Taking the edge off your fun by recounting their 'martyr' acts** – *'Sounds like you enjoyed the great weather. I spent the weekend shopping and cooking for my mum ... you know she's had a stroke.'/'Have fun. They needed someone to cover Christmas again. Jim's had to go in for an operation.*

He'll be recovering. So I offered – you never know when your own luck will turn.'

10. **Using humour to have a dig** – [Pointing at Daddy] *'Here comes Humpty, run up and catch him before he falls!'/'At last! So did you decide to travel by horse today?'*
11. **Make sarcastic comments** – *'Oh, so you had enough time to spend with her, did you?/'Did you enjoy the scenic route? I thought I might have died of starvation by the time you arrived.'/'So that's being a friend, is it? Very caring of you, I'm sure, discussing my private life with her.'*
12. **Pretending there has been a misunderstanding** – *'I probably misheard. I'm sure I got it wrong ... I thought I heard you say that you can't make Johnnie's first football match after all?'/'Hi, Ian, Jan* [a mutual friend] *told me that she saw you in a restaurant in London with a woman; I said that can't be true – she must have mistaken you for someone else. I knew you were working late because you asked me to pick up the kids as Gina* [Ian's wife] *was working late too.'*
13. **Calling in God's help** – *'God is always watching.'/'In the end, God will judge you.'*

Of course, my lists haven't been able to cover all the clever, manipulative tricks people think of when they want to lay a guilt trip on you. Family, friends and colleagues who know us well will personalise their techniques. This means that only the person being tripped knows what they really mean. Others who are hearing what has been said or done may say, *'Sounds like she just wants to make sure you are okay,'* or *'He was only pulling your leg.'* It is important, therefore, to identify the typical and personalised phrases that you know are used to press your particular buttons.

EXERCISE: SPOTTING GUILT-TRIPPING BEFORE IT TRAPS

- Read the list above and note down or mark the types that you recognise.
- Where I have given examples, add one or two of your own that people in your life might use.
- Choose three to watch out for during the next two or three weeks. Note them. You can deal with the others later. If you don't go step by step you will start seeing guilt-tripping everywhere!

Another good way to build your resistance to being tripped is to compose and learn a personal list of rights. These should be related to your own Achilles' heel, which is usually an issue that you already feel some guilt about. This could be a non-priority issue that you have decided to live with for the present.

EXERCISE: IDENTIFYING MY RIGHTS

Read the example list below. Cross out the ones that don't apply to you and add your own. Alternatively do a completely new list that has more meaning for you.

As long as I don't knowingly hurt others or infringe their liberties, I have:

- the right to make moral, lifestyle or relationship choices that are unusual;
- the right to be young;
- the right to be old;
- the right to be clever;

- the right to my own cultural preferences;
- the right to be religious;
- the right to bring up children our way;
- the right to choose not to have children, now or never;
- the right to choose the work I want or need;
- the right to spend my money how I wish;
- the right to eat the way that suits me;
- the right to have different sexual preferences;
- the right to choose how to deal with my own health.

....

....

....

....

....

....

Finally, you can prepare some assertive responses to the person who is guilt-tripping you. The people who do this usually have some personal emotional issue that is driving them. This could be based in feelings such as anger, jealousy, low self-esteem, fear or loneliness. We may guess, or even know, what that is. But you need to remember that whatever it may be it is not relevant. Our goal here is to deal assertively and sensitively with the guilt-tripping behaviour. This is not the time to rescue the tripper from whatever difficulty they may be suffering. The fact that they are suffering does not give them the right to make you suffer with guilt. If you truly want to help them with their issue, choose another day when you have time to give and when you are both feeling less emotionally raw.

Your priority now is self-protection. You need to break their guilt-tripping habit by changing the way <u>you</u> respond. If they are continually guilt-tripping you, they are doing so because your response is giving them some satisfaction. No one can guilt-trip you without your cooperation.

How to respond assertively when being guilt-tripped

There are four dos and four don'ts to bear in mind when responding to being guilt-tripped:

The four dos

✓ Be calm.
✓ Be polite.
✓ Be brief.
✓ Be focused only on the guilt-tripping behaviour.

The four don'ts

✗ No sarcasm.
✗ No revenge guilt-tripping (however tempting!).
✗ No responding to questions.
✗ No responding to irrelevant comments.

To illustrate how you can do this in practice, I will use as examples a few of the 13 common guilt-tripping behaviours that I listed on pages 154–156. This is how you could respond:

Example 1

- Here's some freshly baked ginger bites ... I know you're busy today, but could you just run me down to the station? Taxis are so expensive nowadays.

➘ Thank you – they smell delicious, but I can't run you down to the station today.

- You must be able to spare five minutes. What are you doing?

➘ I just can't run you down today.
[Note: Did not comment on 'taxis are so expensive', did not become aggressive and say, 'I don't have to explain my life to you,' and did not give in!]

Example 6

- I don't have a rich dad like you; I thought you wouldn't mind me borrowing a tenner.

➘ I have the right to my own money. Please return that tenner.
[Note: Ignored the irrelevant snipe at his privileged background, and asked directly for the return of the tenner.]

Example 7

- Your organic food may taste better, but it costs a bomb. Most people can't afford it.

➘ Yes, it is expensive, but that's how I choose to spend my money.
[Note: Did not comment on the guilt-tripper saying 'most people can't afford it'.]

Example 11

- So that's being a friend, is it? Very caring of you, I'm sure, discussing my private life with her.

➘ I am sorry you are upset. No names were mentioned, as I said before. I thought she might have some helpful ideas.
[Note: Empathised and just simply repeated that confidentiality was not breached.]

Example 12

- Jan [a mutual friend] told me that she saw you in a restaurant in London with a woman; I said that can't be true – she must have mistaken you for someone else. I knew you were working late because you asked me to pick up the kids as Gina [Ian's wife] was working late too.

➘ Thank you for picking up the kids. I am not going to comment on Jan's gossip.
[Note: Did not comment on the 'misunderstanding' manipulation, and ignored the guilt-tripping hidden question, i.e. 'Were you two-timing your wife?']

Guilt-trips frequently induce not just strong feelings of guilt, but equally strong feelings of resentment toward the manipulator.

DR GUY WINCH, *PSYCHOLOGY TODAY*, MAY 2013

EXERCISE: RESPONDING TO GUILT-TRIPPING BEHAVIOUR

- Select some other examples of guilt-tripping comments from my list on pages 154–156. Create a concise, polite, assertive response. Add one or two of your own real-life examples.
- Practise saying all the responses out loud. Preferably ask for some help from a friend and do a role-play. Other people can often spot an aggressive dig that we might have understandably slipped in without realising. (There aren't many people who wouldn't welcome an opportunity to brush up their skills in this area. It's a tough call for all of us.)
- Refresh your Broken Record skills (see page 119), because you may need to repeat your core message over and over again. Guilt-tripping is often a habit of a lifetime and could take some time to break.
- Finally, try not to engage in guilt-tripping behaviour yourself. As I said earlier, this is so tempting to do because revenge is an automatic reaction when we feel we have been disempowered. (And, yes, guilt-tripping is a way of depowering others!) Ask your good friends to tell you if you ever engage in this behaviour yourself. Explain that sometimes you may not realise that you have used this kind of manipulative behaviour. If it has been used on you for years, you would have to be a saint not to have picked up a little of the habit. You certainly don't want your friends to be building up feelings of resentment towards you.

Let me assure you that once you have gained more control over guilt-tripping there will be light and laughter at the end of the tunnel. Humour is very curative for out-of-date emotional baggage. Within a close, trusting personal relationship, pushing each other's guilt buttons can become a fun, competitive game. My husband and I play it almost every day. I love it because, perhaps unsurprisingly, I am usually the winner! But on a more serious note, I also know this humorous teasing has been a way of helping us both finally gain some healthy perspective on our painful guilt issues.

Finally, remember, if you have a sensitive conscience, there will always be someone who will attempt to guilt-trip you. Many more people will respect and love you because you have this wonderful quality.

CHAPTER 7

Tips for the Nine Problematic Guilts

Suppressed guilt

As I suggested earlier in Chapter 2, this guilt is almost always better out than in. Much of the advice I have already given in this book should prove useful for dealing with it. If you have any of this guilt hiding within you, before you start it is important to think and plan carefully how you will go about 'outing' it.

How long you will need to put aside to do this will depend on how much guilt you feel and how long you have been suppressing it. It is hard to predict how much time you will actually need to factor in, but I suggest that you allow as much time as you can. Here's what you will need to do:

1. Think carefully about who to talk to and how to ask them (see my guidelines below).
2. Script out (at least roughly) what you want to say. (The section on scripting on page 91 will help.)
3. Use the DREAM Repair Kit to analyse your guilt (see Chapter 5).
4. Do an action plan (Chapter 9, Guilt into Goals, will help) and talk it over with your friend. You could also show them your DREAM analysis if you would value their comments.

5. Put your plan into action.
6. Reward yourself. (This is crucial for renewing your self-confidence. What you will have done is extremely stressful. It is also very courageous and deserves a reward!)

I hope that this long list hasn't put you off. I promise it will be worth your while to do this well. It will affect how you manage guilt in the future. Suppressed guilt can turn into disguised guilt. If that does happen, your problem will be much more difficult to deal with, partly because it could have already hurt you and your relationships, and possibly hurt others as well. Once you have learned and practised this new approach, it will become a habit and the process will take much less time.

Ideally, it is good to have some help. Hopefully this could be one of your friends. If not, you may need to talk to a counsellor or therapist. His or her first role will be that of being your listener. To do that well requires some skill and for the listener to possess certain qualities. Whomever you decide to open up to, try to ascertain whether they have these qualities:

1. Select someone to whom you can tell your story

Your listener will need to:

- be non-judgemental enough to care about you even though you are not perfect;
- truly believe that people can change and improve themselves;
- be able to listen without needing to constantly jump in and reassure and rescue you, or perhaps try to convince you that you shouldn't feel guilty!
- have the ability to empathise without needing to use up your whole time together to tell you their story about their guilt;
- be confident enough to be able to tell you that they don't want to help after all. (Your story might press uncomfortable buttons for them, or they might feel that supporting you will be too time-consuming or emotionally difficult.)
- be unlikely to push you into following their advice (rather than letting you work out your own way of dealing with it);

- have a practical and positive approach to problem solving and will support you in planning how to move on to your next step.

2. Do a DREAM analysis

This helps you prepare yourself before you approach other people who may have been involved or you may have hurt. It will also help to calm you down. You will feel extra guilty because you have been suppressing your wrongdoing, so you will need to take care when assessing your true responsibility.

3. Confess and apologise to the victim

Be aware that your victim and any supporters they may have will be very shocked and possibly angry. If that is the case, don't expect to resolve the situation in one meeting. If, in their anger, they try to push you into immediate action, use a Broken Record statement (see page 119) to postpone further discussion. Do the same if you find that your own feelings are running high or you realise that you need to speak to other people before discussing the matter further. Stay calm and just repeat your key phrase over and over again until they accept it.

For example (the Broken Record phrase is in bold):

A – *I can understand why you are so upset. I am very sorry to have done this and also not to have told you earlier. But I don't think it is a good idea to* ***discuss it further right now****. I'll get back to you tomorrow/next week.*

B – *No, I want you to tell me right now what you are going to do about it.*

A – *I really don't think it is a good idea to* ***discuss it further now****.*

B – *We have waited long enough to get to the bottom of this ... I could speak to your boss, you know.*

A – *I promise I will get back to you tomorrow, but I am not going to* ***discuss it further now****.*

4. Practice the DREAM script you prepared earlier for making amends

This is where your supportive friend can really help. Role-playing using your script is the best way to build your confidence. If you can't do this, practise saying it a few times in front of a mirror.

5. Reward yourself after you have had your follow-up discussion

Remember why this is important? You have been doing your best to deal with one of the most difficult kinds of guilt and deserve a reward. But also remember that rewards help to reinforce new good habits, which is exactly what you are trying to do.

Disguised guilt

This is not, of course, a guilt that is easy to spot in yourself. But if you do become aware of it, you can take steps to ensure that in future the signs are noticed earlier rather than later. As I said in Chapter 2, this kind of guilt has many different disguises, so it is important that such a list of warning signals is personalised. I suggest you take the following steps to do this:

1. Compile a list of early warning signals, preferably with the help of an empathic person who knows you well. The signals can vary enormously, but common examples of behaviours that may indicate disguised guilt are: drinking more alcohol than usual/starting to smoke again/overworking/cleaning more than is necessary/triple checking/snapping at people/oversleeping/becoming cynical/becoming less or much more sociable.

2. Give copies of this personal list to someone whom you trust and who sees you often in your everyday life. This could be a family member (including an older child), friend or trusted colleague. Explain that entries on the list may or may not be signs of disguised guilt, but you would prefer to be alerted to them anyway, as the signals are unwanted behaviour. Also point out that it is important they record some specific details. Explain that this is because you may well deny the behaviour unless you are shown some recorded details. (This is, after all, the nature of the habit you are attempting to curb.)

You will notice in my list of examples below that I have added a column beside each warning signal for the specific details. Your watchers do not have to record their observations so formally, but they will probably forget the helpful details unless they note them down soon afterwards. You could give them a gift of a little notebook in which to jot down their observations.

3. Ask your watcher to give you feedback. I would suggest that you agree that they do this after they have noticed a certain number of possible signals. It may get tedious and annoying for both of you if this is done every time a signal is noticed.

4. Reflect on what may be causing the resurgence of these signals. Ask yourself if they are merely a result of being overstressed, or if they could be something to do with guilt that is either real, imagined or feared. Use your diary to help trigger memories of what you did and whom you were with during that time period. If you are still puzzled, discuss the problem with a level-headed friend.

And remember that if your warning signals continue to escalate, you can always make an appointment to discuss this with your doctor. Never wait for a crisis to emerge before doing this.

Example of a record of warning signals for disguised guilt

Warning sign	What/When/Where
i. Obsessive cleaning	i. Last Sat (14th) cleaned all day, had 15-min break only for lunch.
ii. Drinking too much	ii. You stayed over four hours in the pub Friday eve and last Tuesday.
iii. Snapping	iii. Snapped at Joe on Sun when he only asked you what the score was.
iv. Overworking	iv. You have brought work home four out of five nights, week starting 20th Sept.
v. Rescuing	v. You insisted on driving Carole to her class when she wanted to walk.

Childhood guilt

Guilt dating back to childhood is a tough nut to crack. But it is certainly not an impossible one. It will just take a little longer to break the bad habits. Ideally it would help to do this self-help work with a friend or two, who are also keen to shift their guilt. But if this is not possible, try to do the work on your own following my four steps.

You can always seek some professional help through your doctor if you find that you need some extra support from a psychotherapist or counsellor who has been trained to work with childhood issues. Bear in mind that some counsellors and most coaches do not have this training.

The four steps in the self-help process are:

1. **Choose one childhood guilt to work on.** It is important in any learning or development work to focus on one

problem at any one time. The first should be one that is not too big or too disruptive.

2. **Assess this guilt** and be clear about how it is impacting on your current life. Use the checklist below to kick-start your thinking.

- Does it stop me from doing anything that I want to do today?
- Is it interfering with any of my key relationships?
- Is it hurting anyone else?
- Is it holding me back in my working life?
- Am I still punishing myself for my wrongdoing?
- Do I still crave forgiveness?
- Have I already made some amends?
- Is there any unhealed emotional hurt attached to this guilt?

3. **Review the suggestions and strategies** in this book and decide which could help with this problem. You could use the contents pages at the front of this book to remind yourself of all the possibilities, or you could use the DREAM Repair Kit (see Chapter 5) to help you decide how much of this guilt you deserve and how you will make amends if you are still harbouring true guilt.
4. Make a **Guilt into Goals** action plan (see Chapter 9).

Guilt isn't always a rational thing, Clio realised. Guilt is a weight that will crush you whether you deserve it or not.

FROM *GIRL AT SEA*, BY AMERICAN NOVELIST MAUREEN JOHNSON

Shameful guilt

Shame is a soul-eating emotion.

C. J. JUNG, SWISS FOUNDER OF ANALYTICAL PSYCHOTHERAPY

Shameful guilt, as I said in Chapter 2, is usually the kind that is the most difficult to shift. Recently I heard an interview with Monica Lewinsky, who had an affair with President Clinton when she was in her early twenties. She was viciously shamed by the media across the world for many years. (Of course, she had done something wrong and did admit her guilt, but she was his employee and only 22 years old, whereas he, at the time, was probably the most powerful man in the world!) After staying silent and out of the public eye for ten years, Monica has started to talk publicly about the effect this shaming had on her and her family. Whatever her motives for doing this may be, it seems that she has learned the hard way just how devastating shaming can be if your personality is still in the process of forming. She said: *'If you haven't figured out who you are, it's hard not to accept the horrible image of you created by others.'*

Monica Lewinsky's words illustrate the central issue that is at the heart of shameful guilt. It strikes at the very essence of your self-image. It can therefore only be repaired by doing some basic therapeutic work to rebuild your self-esteem and confidence. You have to dig deep inside yourself to find out who you really are and want to be. And then, very importantly, you have to prove to yourself by your actions that you can be that person. Only then can you have enough self-belief and respect to ensure that you have a life that will make you both happy and proud.

So if this is a type of guilt from which you suffer regularly, you will usually need to do some serious self-reflection and character rebuilding before you can rid yourself of shameful guilt. When you do start to look at the root causes of this problem you may find, as many people do, that you have a history of being repeatedly told, *'You should be ashamed of yourself,'* whenever you did anything wrong. As the people making these judgements of you were either your elders or 'superiors', or people whom you loved or respected, you would have believed them and duly felt ashamed. This is how the habit of adding shame to guilt is usually developed. As you grew up you wouldn't have needed others to shame you because you would have become adept at shaming yourself.

To help you break this habit, I have devised a simple five-step SHAME strategy, which you can use as a guide to kick you into action when you feel shameful guilt. It will remind you to deal first with the shame before you try to resolve the guilt issue. If you do this regularly for a while, and continue to keep your self-esteem boosted, you will eradicate this self-destructive shame habit. Because we are human, we all feel guilt from time to time. But we don't have to make that task more than doubly hard by adding shame to it.

The SHAME strategy

1. **S**eparate the shame from the guilt.
2. **H**eal the shame.
3 **A**nalyse the guilt.
4. **M**ake amends.
5. **E**mpower yourself.

Let me add some 'how-to' flesh to the bones of these five stages.

1. Separate the shame from the guilt

Re-read my introduction to shameful guilt in Chapter 2 (page 40) to remind yourself of the differences between the two emotions. Then you can start to examine your self-shaming behaviours.

a) Note the wrongdoing, e.g. *'I had an affair.'/'I lose my temper too often with the children.'/'I don't work as hard as I know I could, that's why I haven't got promoted.'*
b) Note down examples of how you shamed yourself, e.g. **Self-talk**: *'I am just like my father – a selfish misogynist by nature – that's why I am now sleeping with a married woman.'/'I am a useless, toxic mother – the kids are better off spending as much time with their nan as possible.'/'I am just bone-lazy and a waster. There's no point in trying to get a more interesting job.'* **Behaviour:** *'I didn't talk to anyone about it; I continued to act against my values.'/'I let other people look after the kids.'/'I stopped looking for another job; I acted like a waster – just stuck to the sofa.'*

2. Heal the shame

Use a self-help programme to examine the origins of your shame. Two of my earlier books, *Self-Esteem* and *The Emotional Healing Strategy,* are both guides to dealing with the root as well as the current causes of low self-esteem. Both are easy-to-follow self-help programmes. They can be done on your own but are most beneficial with the occasional input from a friend. They can also be worked through in a small self-help group. The 'group' can have as few as two members, but often works best if there are a few more people. I wouldn't advise having more than eight in a group for working on this kind of issue. It does require that a good deal of trust is built up within the group and that everyone has a chance to participate.

If you haven't time to do this kind of programme right now, look at my tips for boosting your self-esteem on page 54 and these will at least boost you enough to nudge you into some kind of action. You can also find many more tips in my books *The Self-Esteem Bible* and *101 Morale Boosters.*

3. Analyse the guilt

After your self-esteem has been restored, use the DREAM Repair Kit to help identify your share of the responsibility and what to do about it (see Chapter 5).

4. Make amends

a) Apologise effectively – see page 90 for how to do this.
b) Make what amends you can at the moment. Note down also what you may be able to do later (perhaps when the root causes of your shame habit have been more fully repaired).

5. Empower yourself

a) Re-read Chapters 3 and 4 on qualities and life skills. Note down what you need to work on in order to improve your ability to deal with your shameful guilt habits.
b) Decide where you want to start and make an achievable action plan for yourself. This will hopefully include getting some support from a friend to help you keep to your targets. (See the action plan templates in Chapter 9, pages 197–202.)

If, after doing this self-help work, you are still unable to move forward, seek some professional help. And try not to feel ashamed about doing so!

Affluence guilt

This guilt can, of course, become very positive. It ignites philanthropy and social action, which can actually lead to a more just and economically fair distribution of wealth. But if action isn't taken, it leads to apathy, cynicism and low self-esteem.

Here are just a few ways that you can utilise the prod that this guilt can give you. As I have no idea what your personal circumstances are, I have chosen examples of practical action that cost virtually no money and only a minimal amount of time. Reading these should get your own ideas flowing. (Make a note of them before they get lost in the mayhem of everyday life!)

Once we realise that imperfect understanding is the human condition, there is no shame in being wrong, only in failing to correct our mistakes.

GEORGE SOROS, HUNGARIAN BUSINESSMAN AND PHILANTHROPIST

- **Select certain issues.** Don't overwhelm yourself with so many that your contribution, in terms of time and money, feels like a meaningless drop in the ocean.
- **Decide on a realistic contribution** – in terms of money, time or skills you can at present realistically afford.
- **Make an action plan**. Ensure that it has specific goals, which are deadline dated and can be checked.
- **Stay aware and informed.** If you are active on social media, pass on information that could raise awareness of deprivation and hardship. Balance that with more positive information, such as news of money raised for charity and major innovative projects that are making a big difference.
- **Name and shame.** Pass on examples of people and organisations who are, for example, wasting resources, paying

too low wages, etc., but only when you are very sure of your facts. Ian Muir, a senior advisor in business ethics and author of *The Tone from the Top* (Gower Publishing Ltd, 2015), recently reported that companies and local councils are now strengthening their whistleblowing policies by widely publicising the telephone number to ring in confidence.
- **Keep others correctly informed.** If you hear people saying something that you know to be wrong or that could possibly be wrong, be courageous enough to challenge them. For example: *'Those people are not true refugees, they're just scroungers.'* Using a non-aggressive tone, you could say something like: *'I heard an interview that quoted a properly researched survey and the figures were ___. Perhaps you have other information.'*

> **Many who seem to be struggling with adversity are happy; many, amid great affluence, are utterly miserable.**
>
> TACITUS, A ROMAN HISTORIAN

- **Be politically active** – at the very least, find out election dates in good time and schedule in time to vote; keep yourself well informed by listening to or reading both sides of the debate.

Survivor guilt

Nowadays after major disasters most survivors are provided with counselling. Religious organisations and most military organisations have programmes to both commemorate those who have been lost in conflicts and also support the survivors. There are also bereavement counselling services in most countries, often staffed by trained volunteers who may have had similar experiences. By having counselling, you should be able to prevent your feelings of guilt from turning into major illnesses such as Post-Traumatic Stress Disorder (PTSD) and serious depression.

There are, of course, other kinds of survivor guilt that do not involve death. For example, survivors of redundancy programmes. Many enlightened organisations now provide access to counselling for the remaining staff. This is because it is now known that this kind of survivor guilt can affect the remaining staff's morale and motivation.

If you have been a survivor of another kind of major tragedy or serious wrongdoing, such as being a witness to the abuse of someone else, do try to find a counsellor or therapist to help you with your emotions. Never feel that this is something you have to manage on your own.

The majority of survivor guilt, however, is the result of more everyday situations, like losing a relative or a friend. It is one of those kinds of guilt that most people suffering from it know in their heads they need not feel, but they still do. Most will keep it to themselves because they don't think they deserve help. So although, of course, I beg to differ on this point, I think most of you who are reading this book and suffering from this kind of guilt might prefer to try to help yourself. So here are some of my personal tips, which I hope will help you.

- **Give yourself some quality emotional healing.** It is easy to slip back into a grief state when a memory surfaces or you hear a story that triggers empathy in you. I believe that we need to go through five essential stages in order to move on after a personal loss. There are also two other 'bonus' stages to work through if you wish to become super-healed. Take yourself at least through these first three stages, even if you have done them before:

1. Explore what is in your thoughts (particularly about your guilt) by writing about it or talking in confidence to someone. Doing this will stop these thoughts from circling around in your head.
2. Express your feelings by sharing them with an empathic friend and/or releasing your physical tension.
3. Comfort yourself with a nurturing treat or find someone to hug you either physically or metaphorically by giving you a treat. (See my book *The Emotional Healing Strategy* for many more ideas on this subject.)

- **Make anniversaries a pleasure for you** and those around you. You can still cry your heart out as well if you wish, but also try to associate these occasions with beauty and pleasure. Simple ways to do this are buying some flowers, going for a walk in a lovely park or cooking a special meal. In the early years after my daughter's death, I bought a present for myself on each of the anniversaries. I stopped doing this after a while, but we continue to ensure that we have family contact, light candles for Laura and have a quiet, pleasurable day wherever we all are in the world.
- **Keep in contact with people who share your sense of loss** – they don't have to feel the guilt that you feel, but sharing appreciations is comforting.
- **Write a letter to the person or people you are missing** – express your feelings and appreciations. This is particularly important if you were left with many thoughts about what was left unsaid. Like many people, I find jotting down thoughts in a beautiful journal very healing.
- **Create a keepsake box**. Add something whenever you feel the survivor guilt feelings. This could be a poem, a small piece of jewellery or just a small object that can be a symbol of your relationship or your love or concern.
- **When the blues descend, ask a question of the person you lost**. Imagine the answer they would give. I do this from time to time with various people whom I have loved and lost. I always find that I 'hear' a response that encourages and supports me.
- **Compose a confession** if you are still haunted by thoughts of what you didn't do or what you did do that may have hurt them. Put it away somewhere and then, after a week, take your confession out, tear it up and burn or bin it. Then, as soon as you can, do something kind for someone else in your life that you care about. This is a good way of making constructive amends and will help heal your guilt, but any similar idea that would help someone else would do just as well.
- **Change your regret language**. I missed being at my father's bedside when he was dying, and I feel guilty

about the fact that I was not contactable. For a long time I used to think and talk about this regret using negative language such as: *'I feel so bad that I wasn't there in time.'* This made me feel worse and my 'poor me's must have been hard to listen to as well. I decided to try to use more positive-sounding language, such as, *'I would love to have been at his bedside, but I know he would understand the problem. He was himself "out of contact" for much of his life.'* It did, and still does, help. So I experimented with doing the same with my survivor guilt over my daughter's death. And it helped with that as well.

> **The bravest people are not the ones brave enough to die, but the ones brave enough to live, and living is different from surviving.**
>
> ANONYMOUS

- **Give a donation**. I have had a couple of cancer scares recently and, as I often do, I started chatting to people in the waiting room of the hospital. As I left the hospital the first time, I remembered those people and felt a major pang of survivor guilt. After my second scare, I felt the same pang of guilt as I walked past sufferers of the disease, but on this occasion I decided to do something constructive about it. I returned to the reception desk and put a donation into the cancer charity box. A minor act, but it did help me and there was nothing else I could realistically do to help the less fortunate people I had met.

Parental guilt

There is a wealth of parenting books and websites now available to help you with this guilt. The issue is such a common subject of informal debate among parents and is a favourite topic for journalists. Most of the strategies I have already introduced in this book should be useful. However, as a parent who has suffered so much with this kind of guilt myself, I can't resist sharing a few of my own personal tips.

Remember, perfect parents aren't perfect

They can produce very mixed-up, unhappy people, as this quote from the actress Natalie Wood, who struggled with depressive episodes in her adult life, illustrates:

I saw my parents as gods whose every wish must be obeyed or I would suffer the penalty of anguish and guilt.

NATALIE WOOD, AMERICAN ACTRESS

Look for meaningful wisdom on internet discussion forums and then share your own

This was a facility that was unknown to pre-internet parents such as myself. I often felt so alone in a small rural town. I was one of the very few mums in my area who worked and I was at least ten years older than everyone else in parenting meetings. It would have been so comforting and enlightening to read personal stories and reflections such as these:

I remember a time when our son was having difficulties in school. His teacher called about his behaviour and my first reaction was to get angry and defensive and blame myself. But my husband was so clear when he said, 'This is not about you, Esther – it's about our son.' This was helpful in prompting me to change and not take what was happening personally. I needed to remove myself from the picture and focus on my child and what he needed.

I find it painful to see my children struggle with the amount of work they need to do nowadays. I often give in. Have you ever cleaned your child's room, even though he was supposed to do it – and then felt guilty? It can be so much easier to take on our kids' mistakes than to hold them responsible.

Helping others with their guilt will help you. (This is, of course, partly why I am writing this book!)

Remind yourself that sibling spats are normal and not your fault

Parents who are easily tripped into guilt see these arguments as their failure. This is often the case if their own childhood was problematic, and giving their children a happy and harmonious childhood is one of their most cherished goals.

Sibling quarrels teach your children so much about sharing, caring, conflict resolution and the differences between each individual human being. Try to only intervene when bullying or other truly bad behaviour is taking place. When my daughters were in their late teens, I overheard them laughing in an affectionate way about the spats they'd had in their childhood. As I listened, I recalled all the angst and guilt these quarrels had so unnecessarily aroused in me. If only I had been a little wiser at the time!

If you get on better with one, just deal with it

In the real world, this is normal. It is a romantic parental myth that parents can have the same relationship with each of their children. I have heard too many parents protest that they bend over backwards to treat all their children exactly the same. Of course, they fear that this isn't the truth and so are riddled, in secret, with guilt. It can take some time to help them face this reality. They feel as though they have been committing a major parental sin.

If a genetic fluke has made you more in tune with one or more of your children, don't deny it – deal with it. Ensure that you spend quality one-to-one time with the children who are less compatible with your temperament and interests. Spend time with them doing what they like to do. Tell them that you love the fact that they are different from you. Give them examples of how they have opened your eyes to new worlds and how you appreciate (or would appreciate) their help with your weak areas (for example, to be more analytical/become emotionally expressive or creative/to appreciate certain music or sports activities or scientific exploration, etc.).

You can also try to find other adults in or outside the family who may happily spend time with your child doing something together that might bore you to death. If your child's obvious joy at sharing such a mutually enjoyable time with another adult makes you feel insecure or a tiny bit jealous, just deal with that, too! This is going to be a feeling that you will have many more times in your life, and that again is quite natural. Just give yourself a nurturing treat in recompense and move on.

If you are part of a blended family, express your pride and joy in being so

Contact the UK National Step-family Association, or one that is similar, if you need any support and advice. Do this preferably before the issue or dilemma becomes a problem. Remember, these organisations exist because other people share your concerns. And they want to share the wisdom they have accumulated through their difficult experiences. If you later do so yourself, this will help heal any guilt you may be experiencing right now.

> **While children themselves are increasingly relaxed about being in a 'reconstituted' family – partly because of the rise in levels of divorce and remarriage – adults are still building a 'wall of silence' around the issue.**
>
> UK NATIONAL STEP-FAMILY ASSOCIATION

If you have one child that needs you more, explain why to any siblings

This is something I cannot recall doing until it was too late. A few weeks before my younger daughter's death, I talked to my older daughter about just this issue. She was home from her university in France for Christmas. I said that I was aware that I had had to prioritise looking after her sister, Laura, for quite some time because she had been depressed after quitting her university course. But now that Laura was settled with a new course, I wanted to make it up to her sister and support her more. I knew that she was struggling to settle in her accommodation and told her that I planned to visit her in France very soon.

Of course, it was not my fault that this didn't happen, but that did not stop me feeling very guilty. (Parental guilt is often irrational, as you may know.) Over twenty years later, I still feel physical pangs of regret for not having had this conversation with her earlier.

Avoid expressing your parental guilt in front of the children

They don't need your burden as well as the inevitable amount of guilt they will collect for themselves from the outside world. Ask your co-parent or a friend to tell you if you do this. Then, if this guilt is rational, be a good role model and show your children how you can apologise and make amends. If you know your guilt is irrational, tell them that it is so. If they are old enough, use this opportunity to explain why we can all sometimes feel this way, even when we haven't actually done anything wrong.

Carer's guilt

Early in my career, when I was working for a mental-health charity, I had a client who was suffering from chronic depression. She had shared with me her day-to-day life looking after her very old mother. Not only was her life physically exhausting, she was also extremely lonely and felt very guilty about her feelings of despair and resentment. She had willingly given up her successful career as a teacher to look after her mother, and had promised her that she would never let her enter a home. Now she was feeling very sorry for herself and hated the person she had become.

Caring for carers was certainly not a subject I knew anything about at that time, even though I was a fully trained psychiatric social worker. The subject was just not on our curriculum. After researching the services available to carers I was shocked to find that there was so little support available. Our organisation, being a charity, had no spare funds, but we did have a room. So I started a self-help group and asked my client to help me with the publicity and administration.

Very soon this was well attended and made a big difference to people's lives. Not only did they find friends, they found people who were prepared to offer each other practical help and relief. I contributed by doing confidence and assertiveness training with them to help them ask more effectively for what they needed. Social Services were so impressed by the group that they began to give it funding. And, as you might have guessed, another reward for me was that my client's depression lifted.

Nowadays, there are many more organisations supporting people who are carers, though certainly not everywhere. Today, thankfully, you will find support groups in most large towns, and there are very helpful internet forums as well. However, I understand that there are still many unsupported carers for people suffering with different issues. Guilt, I am told, is one of the biggest among these.

So if you are a carer and are not receiving the support you need, why not try the following:

- **Set up your own self-help support group.** I told my story to illustrate just how easy this can be to do. All you need is the use of a sitting room for a couple of hours a week. A kettle would, of course, be an added bonus! Most local government authorities can now provide administrative support for new self-help groups. They can usually advise you on how to set up the group and how to deal with the problems that sometimes arise. My own suggestions are:

1. **Rotate the leadership** of the group, making the change about every month between the people who are willing to do it. Leaders need to ensure that everyone has time to share and make their suggestions. They also need to stop people talking over each other (no easy task!).
2. **Divide the session up** into supportive sharing during the first half, then a break for refreshments, followed by self-help exercises. Let members take it in turns to lead an exercise, such as the ones in this book. There are also many other kinds of exercises in my other self-help books. Certainly confidence and self-esteem building would be useful, as would assertiveness training and dealing with

guilt. If you publicise the list of subjects you will be covering in the exercise session, you will have no problem attracting people.

3. **Finish with a goal-setting session.** This will really help move people forward positively and stop the group from becoming overwhelmed by too much sharing of depressing stories.

• • •

- **Search the internet for advice.** When doing so, remember that most issues carers have are very similar (e.g. how to make a good case for a grant; how to assert yourself with authority figures; how to say 'No'; where to find respite care; family issues, etc.). Have a look at the Alzheimer's Society website: www.alzheimers.org.uk. They have excellent factsheets and advice that would be very helpful for all kinds of carers. One of their factsheets is called Dealing with Guilt and is very good. Another website to look out for is Carers UK's: http://www.carersuk.org/. This has an excellent online forum and very good advice on practical issues such as finance and support. The organisation also campaigns on behalf of all carers.

> **One person caring about another represents life's greatest value.**
>
> JIM ROHN, AMERICAN ENTREPRENEUR AND MOTIVATIONAL AUTHOR

Religious guilt

Maybe religion is not the solution to guilt after all. Maybe, if the truth were known, we'd find that religion and guilt are sweethearts. After all, wherever you find one, the other will usually be buzzing nearby like some fat, annoying housefly.

J. MICHAEL FEAZELL, *CHRISTIAN ODYSSEY* MAGAZINE, 2006

When I was doing the research for this book, I found that the vast majority of other books on guilt were ones written by authors who had a religious perspective on the subject. So for this type of guilt there is already a good deal of help around. But then, I also found this quote, so maybe there is still some way to go in this field.

> **Sadly, we do a much better job of making people feel guilty than we do of delivering them from the guilt we create. We need to confess this and change our ways.**
>
> TONY CAMPOLO, AMERICAN CLERGYMAN

Certainly, from my own clinical experience, it does appear to be a contemporary problem. And it is undoubtedly troubling many people, particularly in multicultural cities. The cases I encounter centre mainly around family issues, with the occasional work dilemma also proving a challenge. These few tips reflect my limited experience.

Clarify your own personal values

Some of these may well be in line with your religious values, but some may clash and produce dilemmas for you. See the section on moral intelligence in Chapter 4.

Ask 'what if' questions

You can do this quite casually in everyday interactions with friends by posing questions that will stimulate debate around your dilemmas. For example:

- What if your daughter wanted to marry someone from a different faith and was insisting that your grandchildren were brought up in that faith, how would you feel?
- What if you were offered a great job with double your salary but they wouldn't allow you to take time off for prayers, would you accept?
- What if you fell in love with someone who had very different religious views from you?
- What if your teenage son simply point blank refuses to go to worship/prayers with the rest of the family?

- What if an important colleague invited you to dinner and you forgot to tell them you don't eat certain foods and that is exactly what has been cooked. What would you do?

Keep your self-esteem topped up

This will help you to stand up for what your conscience is telling you is the right thing to do.

Learn the skill of saying 'No' assertively and sensitively

See Chapter 4. This will help you to avoid religious guilt by making you less vulnerable to being 'seduced' by temptations and pushy people.

Increase your empathy

Re-read my discussion in Chapter 3 on this personal quality and try out some of my tips for strengthening it. Empathy will help you to understand much more accurately people with another religious viewpoint. It does not mean that you will have to change your own beliefs and religious practices, but you may have to find a way of cooperating or just living with a new multicultural reality.

All religions are the same: religion is basically guilt, with different holidays.

CATHY LADMAN, AMERICAN COMEDIAN

CHAPTER 8

How to Help Others with Their Guilt

Admitting to guilt is never easy for anyone, unless of course you are another Gandhi! For some people it can feel virtually impossible, even if they know it would help them to do so. I hope that when you have learned to manage guilt better yourself you will be motivated to use your learning to help others.

> **Confession of errors is like a broom that sweeps away the dirt and leaves the surface brighter and clearer. I feel stronger for confession.**
>
> MOHANDAS GANDHI, LEADER OF THE INDIAN INDEPENDENCE MOVEMENT

Some of you may be reading this book because you already know someone or some people you want to help. If so, I hope it has already given you many ideas about how to do this. Here are a few more tips and reminders that I hope will also be useful.

Be an inspirational role model

Keep doing the exercises and practising the techniques in this book and you will be one! This truly is the very best way of influencing anyone.

Demonstrate openly how to cope well with your own guilt

Talk about your mistakes and wrongdoings. Obviously, I am not suggesting that you publish these in the press or on social media, but you can do this within your family and among your close friends, and to a limited extent with colleagues. Make clear what you are doing when you are making amends.

Encourage others to be open about their guilt

First, you may need to spot the signs that it could be lurking inside someone. Watch out for those listed below. They are often seen when someone is trying to hide their guilt as they tell a cover-up story. But remember that one or two of these signs may indicate nothing at all. You need to look for a few.

Possible signals that inner guilt is being covered up

- Movement of the head even before talking.
- Changes in breathing – it may gradually quicken and then the person may visibly take a deep breath to calm themselves down.
- Standing very still and staring.
- Fidgeting fingers or shuffling feet.
- Repeating phrases or words over and over again.
- Covering the mouth or throat.
- Giving more information than is needed.
- Using an impersonal tone.
- Using an aggressive tone as you persist with questions.

How to talk to someone who may want to confess

Let's assume you have heard or seen something that has made you wonder if a person may be suppressing some guilt. You have also noticed that he or she seems to have changed somewhat or is not happy. You decide there is nothing to lose by carefully trying to help.

- **Start with non-threatening, open questions** on a small-talk subject, such as *'How was your weekend?'*
- **Gradually ask more specific questions, but still safe ones** that will encourage them to open up a bit more about themselves, e.g. *'So, anything you enjoyed today? ... 'Oh, the science class. So that's your favourite, is it?' ... 'Is it the experiments you like or the theory?'*
- **Ask a general question about their welfare** – e.g. *'So how are doing at the moment? I thought you were looking a bit down the other day.'/'You don't seem your normal self these days. Are you okay?'*
- **Back off if you get blocked the first time.** Instead of persisting, give them a reassuring compliment and an invitation to talk at another time. For example: *'We've been friends for five years now and I think you are a great guy, so if you did ever want to talk to me about something, please feel free. Anyway, we should have a beer together some time.'* They will have taken the hint that you have guessed that there may be something hidden. Trust that the guilt will then do its work and make them feel uncomfortable. The more discomfort it brings, the more likely they are to open up.
- **Arrange to meet or bump into each other in a quiet place.** If this feels a little manipulative, just remind yourself that your moral compass is taking you in the right direction. Even if you have to turn back, you should have done no harm. Keep this next meeting on safe subjects. But look out for body signals, especially ones that may be telling you he or she is beginning to feel more at ease with you (such as the uncrossing of limbs, sitting back, relaxed facial muscles, etc.). You can then move further on at your next meeting.
- **Bring up the subject area around the suspected guilt in a general way** – a moan or two of your own would do! For example: *'Family life can be tough sometimes, don't you think?'/'Roger* [your mutual boss] *is a hard nut, isn't he? He expects perfection – as though that is possible for anyone in this job. But then his boss is no better. It's the company culture – they say their door is ever open, but they don't often walk the talk.'*

- **When and if they start telling their guilt story, make sure you gag yourself.** Softly say fillers like *'umh', 'it's okay' and 'so ...'* if they need some encouragement.
- **Sit silently through pauses** – or if they get completely stuck, using a gentle tentative tone, say something like: *'I have the feeling you want to say more or that some things are hard to talk about – I know that feeling.'*
- **Share something about yourself** without asking a question. For example: *'About 10 years ago I was at a very low ebb and I'd got myself into a mess. I just couldn't talk about it for a long time and became more and more stressed out as a result. When I did eventually speak out it was such a relief.'*
- **Don't play detective.** I love watching TV dramas and am fascinated by the techniques they use in interviews (apart from the violent kind, of course). Resist the temptation to try to trip them up into confessing. You are not an interrogator of criminals. Your role is just that of a patient friend who shows concern and compassion. If you stick to that role, they are more likely to take the opportunity to confess. If they don't do that now, they may do it later. That's a very common pattern.
- **If they do open up, stay in your comfort zone** – don't get side-tracked into trying to solve their 'big' problem around their wrongdoing. Stick with the guilt issue. Share what you found helpful in solving yours. That may or may not include telling them about this brilliant book you read about guilt!

Helping children with their guilt

- **Start early but not too early.** It is difficult to be specific about what age this should be, but as I indicated in Chapter 1 it is unlikely to be before they are three years old. The best guide is to look for when they have begun to empathise and show compassion.
- **Take great care not to add shame to their guilt.** This is so easy to do, even when we know it is wrong. It is still very

commonly done and may be hard-wired into your brain if adults did this to you when you were young. (Re-read the section on shameful guilt in Chapter 2. You can easily adapt most of the advice to suit the age of your child.)

Deal with bad behaviour in two stages

Obviously the age of your child will determine how you put these stages into practice. Don't try to include the Step 2 tasks immediately after the wrongdoing. Children won't be emotionally ready to listen.

Step 1: Immediate response

1. **Stop** – the behaviour immediately.
2. **Label** – it, e.g. you hurt someone/used something without asking/stole something, etc.
3. **Judge** – say that behaviour is wrong.
4. **Apology** – insist they make one now, however grudgingly.
5. **Empathy** – ask them to imagine how they would feel if they were the victim.

Step 2: Later discussion

1. **Discuss** – later, when you are both calmer. Choose a quiet spot.
2. **Apologise** – if you didn't handle the situation perfectly before (we all make mistakes in the heat of the moment!).
3. **Guilt** – use age-appropriate language to help them acknowledge their feelings and explain how they can deal with it.
4. **Distinguish** – their behaviour from their character.
5. **Reassure** – say something positive about their personality or usual good or kind behaviour.
6. **Consequences** – help them see the potential negative consequences of repeating that same kind of behaviour.

7. Amends – give them ideas, e.g. draw a card, let the person they hurt play with their best toy or borrow something, give chocolates, etc.

8. Self-esteem – give them a hug, express confidence and say you know that they have learned from the experience.

Treat bullying even more seriously

Distinguish it from less harmful behaviour by perhaps withdrawing a precious privilege for a period of time. Explain why. Cyber-bullying is apparently increasing. Children often don't realise the consequences of joining in with others who are doing it. Be sure that they understand what bullying is.

Bullying is behaviour that is:
• Repetitive and persistent • Intentionally harmful • Involves an imbalance of power • Causes feelings of distress, fear, loneliness or lack of confidence

It includes:
• Name calling and teasing • Taunting • Mocking • Making offensive comments – verbally, by text message, by email or on social-networking sites • Malicious gossip • Stealing • Physical violence • Making threats • Coercion • Isolation from group activities

Seek help if the bullying continues. Most parenting organisations would help you. Family Lives is an example: http://www.familylives.org.uk/. For legal issues in the UK, try Coram Children's Legal Centre: www.childrenslegalcentre.com. Both of these organisations give free advice.

Spare them the memory of any pain you or your spouse experienced during their birth

This is a tip I read long ago but I can't remember where. It immediately reignited guilt. I knew that I had talked to my first daughter about my 48-hour painful labour with her. I had also compared it to that with my second daughter, which by contrast was an easy and beautiful experience. But this prod of guilt has been useful in my work. Since it happened, I have noticed a number of clients sharing their feelings about their mothers' difficult time when they were born. I am not sure how much psychological damage this type of sharing would actually do unless the intention of the parent was to be hurtful. There is unlikely to be any definitive research on the subject. But why not play safe? This would at least avoid the guilt that I experienced at having possibly triggered this feeling in my eldest daughter.

Don't talk about how much tougher your childhood was than theirs

When they are old enough to understand and discuss this, they may question you. Tell them then, if they want to hear.

Instead of shielding them from money difficulties to avoid giving them guilt, let them help

Ask them to do jobs voluntarily that you might otherwise have to pay for, such as cleaning the car, mowing the lawn or babysitting younger siblings. Be very appreciative. Link requests to turn off lights to helping with the finances, and thank them. Turn finding cheaper brands in a supermarket into a helpful game to play. Tell them, or let them count up, how much money they have saved.

Express and deal with your divorce guilt out of their hearing

They have enough of their own feelings of guilt to deal with on this subject.

Absolve them kindly of any blame they don't deserve

Children are egocentric and when they are young they believe they have the power to make you ill, sad, poor or fight with your partner, etc. I know from my professional work that the guilt they feel can trouble them well into their adulthood (even when they know that the feeling is irrational).

Let them overhear you talking positively about them

This is especially helpful if they are shy or have not done as well as expected at something. It is also good to do if there is a big difference in achievement between them and their siblings, friends or even you.

Feel free to use the fear of guilt to deter and motivate

But not until they can understand. Use, of course, in conjunction with other methods.

My parents are really well intended, and I think their way of dealing with things is denial and guilt. Nobody wanted to talk about it. But all I did was blame myself.

TERI HATCHER, AMERICAN ACTRESS AND PRESENTER

CHAPTER 9

Guilt into Goals

You may now be feeling a little overwhelmed by all the information you have received in this book. So now you need to focus on how you can put some of the learning into practical action. Obviously you cannot, or may not need to, do everything that has been suggested in this book. But if you are going to change your way of handling guilt in the future, you have to start by taking some small achievable steps.

Below, you will find the outline of two templates for action plans. The first is a more general one designed to help you put the learning from this book directly into action. It will help you to choose some specific goals to focus on over the next month. You can use another copy of the template for another month or two if you would like to learn more from this book.

The second action plan is for dealing with specific guilt reactions that trouble you in your forthcoming everyday life. Hopefully you will have made photocopies or saved a file on your computer so it will be ready to use whenever you need it.

In order to make your task more achievable, I have narrowed down the choices for your focus. If you give yourself too many goals, you are less likely to achieve them and will become demotivated.

I have also asked you to show your action plan to someone who will check out your progress and hopefully support you. Doing this will increase your chances of success and make the task much more pleasant. But if this is not possible, don't worry. Just do your best – which, as you know, in personal development work is always good enough.

Notice that I have also asked you to name a suitable reward for either completing your goal or for making an excellent effort to do so. Don't skip this reward – it is very important to positively reinforce all your new good habits.

Action plan 1

Applying the learning from *Skip the Guilt Trap* during the next month

1. Which two or three of these ten types of guilt will I think about and observe in myself and others over the next month? If it is another type that is not listed, name it and tick the 'Other' box. (See Chapter 2.)

☐ Positive guilt
☐ Suppressed guilt
☐ Disguised guilt
☐ Childhood guilt
☐ Shameful guilt
☐ Parental guilt
☐ Survivor guilt
☐ Affluence guilt
☐ Carer's guilt
☐ Religious guilt
☐ Other

2. Which two of the four key personal qualities will I choose to improve in order to help me with my guilt? (See Chapter 3.)

☐ Self-esteem
☐ Humility
☐ Trust
☐ Empathy

How will I do that?
Quality 1: ....
....
Quality 2: ....
....
....

3. Which two of the five key life skills do I need to improve? (See Chapter 4.)

☐ Moral intelligence
☐ Rational thinking
☐ Confident communication
☐ Emotional management
☐ Friendship

How will I achieve that?
Skill 1: ....
....
....
Skill 2: ....
....
....
....

4. Which two of my own guilt situations do I choose to use the DREAM Repair Kit on? (See Chapter 5.)
1. ....
....
2. ....
....

5. Which three actions will I take to ensure that I reduce the number of times I am guilt-tripped by others? (See Chapter 6.)
1. ....
....
2. ....
....
3. ....
....

6. Which three actions will I take to improve my ability to help others with their guilt? (See Chapter 8.)

1. ....
....
2. ....
....
3. ....
....

7. What three actions will I take to ensure that I become less generally prone to feeling guilt? (See Chapter 10.)

1. ....
....
2. ....
....
3. ....
....

8. My reward for achieving this goal or making an excellent effort will be:

....
....
....
....

Show this completed action plan to a close friend and ask them to put a date in their diary when they will contact you to see if you have achieved your goals. Put that date in your diary and also here:

....

Signed: ....

Today's date: ....

Action plan 2

Goals for my guilt

1. Describe the situation that triggered the troublesome guilt reaction.

....

....

....

....

2. What kind of guilt is it? (NB: it could be a mixture of different types of guilt.) Tick the types of guilt that apply to this feeling. If it is another type that is not listed, name it and tick the 'Other' box. (See Chapter 2.)

☐ Positive guilt
☐ Suppressed guilt
☐ Disguised guilt
☐ Childhood guilt
☐ Shameful guilt
☐ Parental guilt
☐ Survivor guilt
☐ Affluence guilt
☐ Carer's guilt
☐ Religious guilt
☐ Other

3. What is my long-term goal? (NB: Some guilt reactions cannot be removed altogether, e.g. those that are hard-wired into our brain in our childhood or those that are constantly triggered by, for example, the media or cultural pressures, which cannot be shifted. For these, the long-term goal would be to stop them affecting current behaviour.)

....

....

....

....

What is a realistic date when I can expect to have reached this goal?

....

4. What is my goal for the next week?

....

....

....

....

What will I do to achieve this goal (e.g. using a strategy/developing a quality/improving a skill or something else)?

....

....

....

....

5. What is my goal for a month's time?

....

....

....

....

What will I do to ensure that I achieve this goal?

....

....

....

....

6. My reward for achieving this goal or making an excellent effort will be:

....

....

....

....

Show this completed action plan to a close friend and ask them to put a date in their diary when they will contact you to see if you have achieved your goals. Put that date in your diary and also here:

....

Signed: ....

Today's date: ....

CHAPTER 10

Keeping Yourself Free from Guilt Traps

Once you have cleared away much of your troublesome guilt, it makes sense to try to stop yourself getting caught in any more guilt traps. So I have written some ideas below on how to do this for you to consider for the future. But do read them now, as it is good to always bear them in mind. The list is easy to read and the titles have checklist boxes, so you can use these as a quick way of reminding yourself of what you have learned in this book. Obviously, the more guilt you can avoid the better. As you know, it does drain our confidence and puts added stress on both our bodies and minds.

☐ Maintain your moral compass

Make sure you always have it pointing in an up-to-date direction. It should be the direction that you want to be morally guided towards now, and not where you were heading ten years ago. Use the exercises in Chapter 4 to update your values and personal life rules to fit in with your current life and goals. Do this at least once a year (add it to your New Year resolutions list, perhaps?) and after any major life transition, such as starting on a new career path, getting married, having children, facing the empty nest, dealing with a major illness or bereavement and, of course, retirement.

☐ Boost belief in yourself

Keep your self-esteem topped up, but ensure your humility is in good enough shape to block you from entering the arrogance zone (see pages 56–59). Watch out also for negative self-talk and blaming yourself for every misdeed you can think of.

☐ Keep your skills sharpened

In particular, practise using the strategies in this book. Use them on small, everyday problems that may or may not relate to guilt. Then, when you do need them for guilt, they will be razor sharp. For example, the Broken Record strategy (page 119) and scripting (page 91) are both very helpful when you need to make a complaint. The GEE strategy (page 85) and reframing (page 81) will deal with any moans from yourself or other people. The Don't Get Too Boiling strategy (page 105) will help you keep your cool with any minor frustration such as late trains, friends and colleagues.

☐ Curb unwanted critics

Use the logic of the Three Cs and GEE strategies to outwit them. Learn assertiveness skills to stop them in their tracks. (For more details take a look at my book *Assert Yourself*.)

☐ Replace rumination with written reflection

Writing engages the cognitive areas of the brain and it can help contain the guilt feelings. When guilty thoughts circle around and around in your head, write them down in a notebook or on any piece of paper. Then underneath write: '*I will take action ...*' and add a date and time, and don't forget to enter that date in your diary.

I would suggest that in this later 'session' with yourself you do a quick DREAM analysis (see pages 165–166). This will deal with most of these obsessive thoughts. If not, do a full analysis followed by an action plan when you have time.

If it happens again, just write down the guilty thought and a statement that summarises what is in your action plan. For example: '*I have a plan to deal with this guilt and it includes making amends for my part and taking steps to ensure others deal with their responsibilities.*'/'*I do not have to feel guilty. I am working hard to be a good-enough parent. It would not be good for my children if I were a perfect parent.*'

□ Do your best to blow away guilt

Doing your best might mean that you don't become a saint, but you will be in the company of many stars. Here are just a few to encourage you.

You want to do everything you can in your power to do your best. And, for me, I know I get insane guilt if I go home at the end of the day and don't feel I've done everything I can. If I know I could have done something better, I have this uneasy feeling.

ANDY RODDICK, AMERICAN TENNIS PLAYER

You can only do your best. That's all you can do. And if that is not good enough, it isn't good enough.

IMELDA STAUNTON, BRITISH ACTRESS

Movies are hard to make, and you have to work toward a common ethic and do your best.

ROBERT DE NIRO, AMERICAN ACTOR

Do your best until you know better. Then, when you know better, do better.

MAYA ANGELOU, AMERICAN AUTHOR

□ Confess carefully

Choose the right kind of friend (see Chapter 4) who can listen empathically. If that person can think analytically, they could also help you to do a DREAM analysis and action plan. But remember, sometimes we need the help of two different friends for these two tasks. Good listeners are not always good analysts and vice versa.

☐ Put pen to paper to keep harsh words inside you

I soothe my conscience now with the thought that it is better for hard words to be put on paper than that Mummy should carry them in her heart.

ANNE FRANK, TEENAGE JEWISH GERMAN-BORN DIARIST WRITING WHILE IN HIDING DURING THE SECOND WORLD WAR

I am always amazed at the wisdom that came out of Anne Frank's mind! How did she know at her young age and in her difficult circumstances that writing out what is in your head can also stop you from you from feeling regret and guilt?

Jack Canfield reminds us that this is especially important to remember when we are with children:

Words, especially when yelled in anger, can be very damaging to a child's self-confidence. The child probably already feels bad enough just from seeing the consequences of his or her behaviour. Our sons and daughters don't need more guilt and self-doubt heaped upon their already wounded egos.

JACK CANFIELD, AMERICAN PERSONAL DEVELOPMENT TRAINER AND AUTHOR

But if you do slip up occasionally, remember that a genuine apology and some reparative words will undo the damage.

☐ Burn-out and breakdowns breed guilt

In my profession you meet many people who have burnt themselves out and have mental-health breakdowns. When they reach this state, they are constantly ruminating about what they haven't been able to do and what they should be doing. They are riddled with guilt. They are not feeling proud about all the people they have helped, the long hours they have worked or the hardships they have overcame.

So if you are a rescuer like me by nature or nurture, make sure that you balance your care of others with care of yourself.

☐ Take your templates with you

For at least the next few months take copies of your DREAM Repair Kit and action plan templates around with you. These will help you to focus immediately on doing something constructive with your guilt before it takes a negative hold on you. Don't forget that it isn't the guilt itself that is intrinsically bad, it is the habits that you have being using to manage it that need changing.

☐ Gather some guilt buddies to watch over each other

Weight Watchers works not so much because of its dietary advice, but because its group members support and motivate each other. Breaking any kind of well-entrenched habit is hard, but it is so much easier when you do so in the company of a group. As we live such busy and geographically scattered lives nowadays, this may be easier to do on the internet than face-to-face. You just need a few friends to agree to regularly share their progress over a month or two.

☐ Watch the way you walk

People for whom guilt has been a problem most of their life have a natural tendency to curl up their body. So check that you are walking with your head held high, your shoulders back and your back erect. Pilates exercises will enable you to do this more easily. Adopting this kind of body posture will do wonders for your self-confidence, too.

☐ Say sorry sensibly and sensitively

Say it once if possible, but only twice if you have to. Personalise your empathy when you acknowledge their hurt feelings. For example: *'I know you must have felt very let down as we have been friends for eight years now and you have always been there for me.'/'You must have felt very scared because I am so much bigger than you. I am so very sorry that I frightened you.'/'I am so sorry not to have managed to get the results to you earlier. I know you have your holidays booked so you must have been particularly anxious.'*

☐ Mothball the myths

Here are just a few of the common unhelpful myths about guilt. I am sure you must have at least some of these buzzing around in your head. And maybe you have some others, too.

- You can't help having feelings.
- Guilt is always bad for you.
- Other people can make you feel guilty.
- All you need when you are guilty is forgiveness.
- You can't change your thoughts, even when you know they are irrational.
- Punishment is the only way to deal with guilt.
- You must be stupid to feel guilt when you know it is irrational.
- People who are guilty should be ashamed of themselves.

I am suggesting 'mothballing' because you may not be quite ready to throw out these myths forever. You may first need to prove to yourself that they are indeed myths and not fact.

This mothballing metaphor came to me because I have recently been putting away loads of clothes and adding mothballs to the bags. I am not ready yet to accept that these clothes will never fit me again. The rational part of me is certain that I will be taking them all to charity shops this time next year. But at least when they are out of sight they are out of mind!

So it might help you to write out a list of the myths about guilt that are around in your mind and to then file it away. Choose the particular myths that have been preventing you from dealing with this feeling in the way you would like to. After a year of trying out the ideas in this book, you might be ready to burn that list.

☐ Use art to activate good guilt

On no account brood over your wrongdoing. Rolling in the muck is not the best way of getting clean.

FROM *BRAVE NEW WORLD* BY BRITISH AUTHOR ALDOUS HUXLEY

Creative people of all types often use art to prick the collective conscience of their communities. It is hard to tell what success they have in doing so, but I am fairly certain that they will have helped subdue their own guilty feelings and at least made some people more aware of ethical dilemmas and hypocrisies.

I recently heard an interview with Michael Nyqvist, a star of the 2009 blockbuster film *The Girl with the Dragon Tattoo,* in which he said:

What Stieg Larsson [author of the book *The Girl with the Dragon Tattoo*] was up to – it was the Swedish guilt over World War Two. All of our neighbours had the most terrible experiences with the bad forces, but Sweden didn't.

MICHAEL NYQVIST, SWEDISH ACTOR

This set me thinking of other artists who have used their art in the same way. I could, I am sure, fill a book with these, but here are just a few that leapt into my mind:

- Picasso's painting of the massacre of the people and animals of Guernica, a small rural village in northern Spain. The event took place during the civil war, but the painting has become an iconic anti-war image.
- Ai Weiwei, the Chinese contemporary artist who was imprisoned in 2011 by his government for his dissident activities and now exhibits his conscience-provoking art all over the world.
- Shostakovich's 7th Symphony, which was written as a musical representation of the horrors of the siege of Leningrad during the Second World War. It became an international symbol of resistance to totalitarianism throughout the world.
- John Lennon's song 'Imagine' is an example from the world of popular culture that again has been played internationally.
- Tolstoy's novels *War and Peace* and *Anna Karenina,* which highlighted the injustices of deep social divisions in the Russia of his day before the revolution.

- The giant replica of Marc Quinn's sculpture of a pregnant woman with no arms and truncated legs that was used for the opening of the London 2012 Paralympics.

If you are not a creative artist yourself, you can at least support artists' efforts by talking about them and bringing more people's attention to them and their messages.

☐ Care for your community

On a smaller scale, you may not be able to solve global problems, but you could do something to make a difference in your local community. This could be in line with your special talents or it could be just doing a boring job, such as delivering leaflets about an important issue. I have just received an email from a neighbour about a local mugging and I am grateful for the warning.

☐ Guilt into goals

This could be a motto for yourself as well as being your action-planning guide.

Finally, I hope that you have been inspired by this book to help yourself with your own guilt habits. I also hope that you will find it useful when trying to help others with theirs as well. I wish you lots of luck with the challenge and hope that it makes a difference to your life and brings you more peace of mind.

Try using my variation on the Serenity Prayer below to keep you motivated.

• • •

Accept with composure the guilt you cannot change.
Change with courage what you can.
Celebrate your successes.

Notes

1. K.W. Fischer, P.R. Shaver and P. Carnochan, 'How emotions develop and how they organise development', *Cognition and Emotion*, 4(2), (1990), 81–127.

2. Michael Lewis, PhD, 'The Self-Conscious Emotions', *Encyclopedia of Early Childhood Development*, Institute for the Study of Child Development, UMDNJ–Robert Wood Johnson Medical School, Child Health Institute, USA (September 2011): http://www.child-encyclopedia.com/emotions/according-experts/self-conscious-emotions.

3. Christian Miller, *International Journal of Ethics* 6(2/3), (2010), 231–252.

4. Rebecca L. Schaumberg and Francis J. Flynn, 'Uneasy lies the head that wears the crown: The link between guilt-proneness and leadership', *Journal of Personality and Social Psychology*, 103(2), (August 2012), 327–342: https://www.gsb.stanford.edu/insights/why-feelings-guilt-may-signal-leadership-potential.

Further Help

Please do visit my own website. I write a regular blog, and now that I have written this book I will be including many more posts on the subject of guilt. Most of my blogs do contain exercises designed to strengthen confidence.

http://www.gaellindenfield.com/

Books

Nowadays, as I find that booklists date so quickly and it is so easy to search for them on the internet, I no longer include them. But I have referred to a number of my earlier books, which I do think would be very useful in managing guilt, so I have listed relevant ones below.

Assert Yourself (Thorsons, 2014, 1996)
Super Confidence (Thorsons, 2014, 1996)
Self-Esteem (Thorsons, 2014, 1996)
Managing Anger (Thorsons, 2000, 1996)
Emotional Confidence (Thorsons, 2014, 1997)
Self-Esteem Bible (Element, 2004)
101 Morale Boosters (Piatkus, 2010)

Useful organisations

Below is a list of organisations that could be helpful. I have only included the websites, as telephone numbers and email addresses can become out of date so quickly.

Action on Depression

Scotland's national charity for people affected by depression, offering Living Life to the Full courses, a network of support groups, an online community and an email support service.

http://www.actionondepression.org/

Anxiety UK

Anxiety UK works to relieve and support those living with anxiety disorders by providing information, support and understanding via an extensive range of services, including one-to-one therapy.

https://www.anxietyuk.org.uk/

CALM

Helpline for men at risk of suicide or wishing to talk to someone.

https://www.thecalmzone.net/

Carers UK

Helpline providing advice and information for carers on any issue including benefits, residential care, the Carer's Act and respite care.

http://www.carersuk.org/

Counselling Directory

Counselling Directory aims to be the leading service for providing counselling advice and information, connecting those in distress with the largest support network in the UK.

http://www.counselling-directory.org.uk/

Depression Alliance

A self-help organisation for sufferers of any kind of depression.

http://www.depressionalliance.org/

Gofal

Provides a range of services for people in Wales, including information on common mental-health problems, advice for employers, and training and support.

http://www.gofal.org.uk/

Mind

Provides information for users of mental-health services, carers and other groups on types of mental distress, treatments, therapies and legal matters.

http://www.mind.org.uk/

OCD-UK

A charity that offers support to Obsessive-Compulsive Disorder sufferers with an excellent website full of information.

http://www.ocduk.org/

Samaritans

The Samaritans provide 24-hour, confidential, emotional support for anyone in crisis.
Helpline: 116 123. This number is FREE to call.

http://www.samaritans.org/how-we-can-help-you/contact-us

SANE

SANE services provide practical help, emotional support and specialist information to individuals affected by mental-health problems, their family, friends and carers.

www.sane.org.uk

YoungMinds

Charity committed to improving the emotional well-being and mental health of children and young people.

http://www.youngminds.org.uk/

Acknowledgements

My biggest thank-you goes to Jane Graham-Maw, my wonderful agent. She achieved what I had thought would be an impossible task – to tempt me back into writing another book. I was so sure that I had given up writing forever! Since signing the contract for this book, I have had a number of personal setbacks to deal with, and Jane has been the most supportive agent I could ever have had through these.

My second major thank-you goes, as ever, to my long-suffering husband, Stuart. He has not only willingly taken on his usual role of editing out most of my dyslexic errors, but he has also produced more than his fair share of meals during a period when he, too, was under immense pressure.

A third major thank-you goes to all the people who have shared with me their difficulties with guilt. Your contribution appears somewhere in the book, even if you have been heavily disguised, or your experiences have just helped me to develop my ideas and strategies. I could never have written this book without your help.

I would also like to thank all the people I have quoted in the book. Most of their words are in the public domain on brilliant websites such as Brainy Quotes and Good Reads. These quotes have added valuable insight and inspiration to the book.

Many thanks, too, go to my commissioning editor at HarperCollins, Carolyn Thorne, and her colleagues. You have been a great team to work with and were very understanding when I had to delay delivering the manuscript.